Easy Everyday Keto

Learn Interesting and Easy Keto Recipes to Lose Weight, Eat Tastefully and Restore Your Physical Condition to Live Healthy

By Andrew Shelby

Table of Contents

Introduction

Congratulations on purchasing *Easy Everyday Keto,* and thank you for doing so. I hope you will find plenty of useful information on the ketogenic diet plan and learn how to use it in your menu planning efficiently.

The keto or ketogenic diet is a moderate protein, low-carbohydrate, and high-fat diet plan that can help your body burn the unwanted fat. Over fifty studies have shown its benefits for your health, weight loss, and performance, making it a technique that is recommended by an abundance of doctors. It can assist you in losing excessive body fat without creating those nagging hunger bouts, as indicated in 2016 in the *British Journal of Nutrition.*

The Meaning of Keto

Your body produces ketones, which are small fuel molecules, which act as an alternate fuel source for the body, especially your brain, when your blood sugar (glucose) is in short supply.

If you're eating fewer calories and fewer carbs, your liver will produce ketones from the fat. Your brain will consume tons of energy daily, and it cannot function on fat directly. It can only operate on ketones or glucose. Ketosis is reached as your body enters a metabolic state when your body produces these ketones.

Fasting (not eating anything) is the quickest way to achieve ketosis, but you cannot fast indefinitely. The ketogenic diet, on the other hand, allows you to continue in the state of ketosis.

You have four basic ways to use to ketogenic dieting techniques:

Keto Method #1:The standard ketogenic diet (SKD) consists of moderate protein, high-fat, and is low in carbs. Generally, this diet is considered a low-carbohydrate (5% average), high-fat (75% average), and moderate protein (20%) diet plan. These are average counts and can vary.

Keto Method #2:Workout times will call for the targeted keto diet, which is also called TKD. The process consists of adding additional carbohydrates to the diet plan during the times when you are more active. This is popular with sportsmen and women who are much more active.

Keto Method #3:The cyclical ketogenic diet (CKD) entails a restricted five-day keto diet plan followed by two high-carbohydrate days.

Keto Method #4:The high-protein keto diet is comparable to the standard keto plan (SKD) in all aspects. You will consume more protein. Its ratio is repeatedly noted as maintaining 35% protein, 5% carbs, and 60% fat. (Once again, these are average percentage

Chapter 1: The Ketogenic Diet Explained

Macros Explained

The first step is understanding the macronutrients and how they're calculated.

The macronutrients are the building blocks of food consisting of protein, fat, and carbs.

Maintain your weight with a balance of high fats and low carbs. To achieve weight loss, you will need to reduce your carbohydrate intake. The ketogenic techniques will provide you with the required foods to lose weight and not be hungry. Macros are found in varying amounts, which are measured using grams. For example, <u>fat equals</u> approximately nine calories per gram, protein at four calories, and the carbs at four calories for each gram.

Count The Calories Or The Macros: Which Is Best?

The short of counting calories is that they don't tell the whole story. You can fill up on the 'right' calories, and you may also lose muscle mass. For example, you count one hundred calories of avocado (a fat), which is better than one hundred-calorie cookie (carbs). That is why keto counts the macros (fat, protein, and carbs), not the calories.

Remember This Formula*:* You will need to calculate your net carbs on some of the recipes you discover on the Internet — some list only the total carbs. If that happens, just take the total carbs listed (-) fiber (=) the total net carbs, which is what you need to track for an accurate count so you can remain in ketosis.

The Role of Calories - Fats, Protein,& Carbs

Carbs Needed Daily to Lose Weight

To achieve weight loss, you will need to reduce your carbohydrate intake. You will soon realize the plan will allow you to feel full and satisfied while still losing weight. You simply restrict carb intake, including starches such as bread and pasta, as well as sugars. As a result of the keto diet, you will replace them with fat and protein. Not only will you lose weight, but you will also lower blood pressure, triglycerides, and blood sugar.

What works for one person as a 'low-carb' diet might be too low for another person. It depends on your activity levels, age, body composition, and gender. It may also depend on your metabolic health, food culture, and personal preferences.

If you are more active and have more muscle mass, you can tolerate more carbs versus someone who is sedentary. If people get metabolic syndrome, he/she may become obese or suffer from type II diabetes, whereas the rules change. It is sometimes referred to by scientists as 'carbohydrate intolerance.'

As mentioned, there's no set rule for carb intake. These are some of the basic guidelines to consider as you blaze the path on the ketogenic diet plan, which is effective about 90% of the time:

Moderate Carb Intake: 100-150 Grams Daily
If you are active and lean trying to maintain weight, these are some of the foods to consider:
- Several fruits daily
- All the veggies you can eat
- Healthy starches such as rice, oats, sweet potatoes, and potatoes

50-100 Grams Daily:
- Plenty of veggies
- 2-3 pieces of fruit each day

- Minimal intake of starchy carbs

20-50 Grams Daily:
Losing weight at the rate of 20-50 g. daily quickly falls into this category. If you have diabetes, are obese, or metabolically deranged, this is the plan for you. If you are consuming less than 50 grams daily, your body will achieve a ketosis state which supplies the ketone bodies.

Consider these guidelines:
- Some berries with whipped cream
- Plenty of low-carbohydrate veggies
- Trace carbs from foods including nuts, seeds, and avocados

As you now see, it is essential to experiment and categorize where you fall on the scales before you make any changes. Seek your doctor's advice before changing your eating patterns. In some cases, you could reduce the need for some medications.

The Balance of Exercising & Eating Habits
If you are not eating sufficient food, your body's metabolism will slow down. Research studies indicate that the metabolic rate can drop as much as 15% if you do aerobic exercise more than one hour daily.

Also, eating too little food can have the same results. In this event, over six months, your metabolic rate would drop by about 6%, with a 25% calorie deficit.

For example, if you are 240 pounds, you can receive approximately 2449 calories from fat storage. At 220 pounds, it would be about 11821 calories. You see how it drops.

Against the logic, add some extra fat and protein to see if it helps. You should also consider a 4-day workout regimen as your maximum training time weekly. Work-out in short intervals any time of the day you feel the need to get moving. You just need fast feet, and high knee lifts to perform your exercises. After all, you are trying to push your heart to its maximum, not your biceps. Give yourself some needed rest.

You must keep track of the macros to ensure your body remains in balance.

Keto Versus Other Famous Diets

The Keto Diet limits the carbohydrate intake at 5% of the energy intake, whereas the low-carb diet plans have no definition. The ketogenic diet is moderate protein, high-fat, and low-carbs. With its limitations of carbs, the diet forces your body to burn the fat for energy (ketosis).

During the introductory stage, the *Atkins diet* is set at roughly 15-30 grams per day of carbs to help promote fat burning instead of using glycogen for energy. Its popularity took a dive when individuals were gaining weight over the long term, getting sick, and increasing their blood lipid profile.

The Paleo diet is a newer trend based on eating, as our ancestors did 10,000 years ago. It consists of eating more fruits and veggies because meat supplies were not always available daily. The foods contain more fiber, omega-3s, vitamins, and minerals. They also had less salt and saturated fats.

Fats aside from meat should come from healthy oils (avocado, macadamia, walnut, olive). The balance of the diet should reflect refined sugar, legumes, potatoes, cereal grains, and dairy.

The South Beach diet operates in phases to help with quick weight loss. The first 14 days is a 'restriction phase' in which you cannot eat, fruit, sugar, alcohol, ice cream, sweets, bread, pasta, rice, potatoes, or baked goods. You will shake your metabolism and halt your sugar dependence, placing your body in fat-burning mode. After two weeks, you can add some of the carbs, including some fruits and brown rice (phase 2). Phase three enters a long-term approach, much like the Mediterranean diet with lean meats, some dairy, fresh fish, and veggies.

Each diet claims to be best for you, so it is up to you to decide!

Hints to Produce Energy From Foods

You need to keep your energy levels high, which means you need a variety of healthy oils and veggies as well as a balance of proteins, carbs, and fats. Since some foods can provide a quick boost that fades quickly, you need to discover ways to reduce cravings between meals. Try one or all of these methods:

- Eat Smaller - More Frequent Meals
- Use Caffeine As A Plus
- Limit Alcohol Intake
- Enjoy Keto Energy Bars

Do You Know What Your Body is Craving?

Your body will tell you what is necessary to keep it going. The message comes to you as a craving. Here are a few cravings with what your body needs and a quick fix for the issue:

Carbs/Bread/Pasta: You need some nitrogen, which can be remedied with some high protein meat.

Chocolate: The carbon, magnesium, and chromium levels are screaming for some spinach, nuts, and seeds, or some broccoli and cheese.

Fatty or Oily Foods: The levels of calcium and chloride need repair with some spinach, broccoli, cheese, or fish.

Salty Foods: Your body is craving silicon. So, grab a few nuts and seeds; just be sure to count them into your daily counts.

Sugary Foods: Several things can trigger the desire for sugar, but typically phosphorous, and tryptophan are the culprits. Have some chicken, beef, lamb, liver, cheese, cauliflower, or broccoli.

The Importance of Drinking Water

You may not know, but water is the main component of your blood. It's essential to carry nutrients to your cells and remove waste products. If you become dehydrated, you will begin showing signs of fatigue. If you enjoy working out (or not), be sure you drink an 8-ounce glass of refreshing water before you begin. It's also vital to have another glassful after you have completed your time on the mats. If you have passed the 30-minute workout, be sure to drink small amounts of refreshing water every 15 minutes to half an hour.

Stock the Fridge

The first area to consider is stocking your refrigerator. Good health depends on using fresh, organic, or raw milk products. Choose from harder cheese items, including mozzarella and cheddar, since they contain fewer carbs. Also, purchase full-dairy items to gain additional calcium and protein. Add non-dairy items, including coconut, almond, or cashew milk. Consider some of these items:

- Brie Cheese - 0.1 grams of net carbs per 1 ounce
- Cheddar or Colby Cheese - 0.4 net carbs per 1 ounce
- Cream cheese - 0.8 net carbs per 2 tablespoons
- Sour cream -1 gram net carb per 1 tablespoon
- Feta Cheese - 1.2 grams net carbs per 1 ounce
- Parmesan cheese - 0.9 per 1 ounce
- Heavy whipping cream - double cream & whipped - 3 grams of net carbs per ½ cup

Understand the difference between ghee (clarified butter) and grass-fed butter. As you begin using your ketogenic recipes, you may notice some of them will have these items listed. You can promote fat loss and retain lean muscle mass using butter. Butter consists of water, milk solids, and butterfat. Ghee, an Indian staple, includes pure butterfat. Therefore, if you have lactose sensitivities, ghee is probably your best choice. The ghee also contains medium-chain fatty acids that assist your immune system and digestion.

Whole Eggs: Search for a local area market for free-range options. You can scramble, fry, boil, or devil eggs up for a picnic or any occasion.

when you finish the 16-day-meal plan, begin to plan your week meals by choosing among the recipes in the book. See our example and insert the recipes you like. Adapt the recipes to your food availability at the moment and fresh seasonal food. You can copy it on a journal if you need.

Purchase Keto-Friendly Fresh Veggies

The values in the list are calculated for the times you don't have a specific recipe to use, so you don't exceed your daily carbohydrate limits. The following list will provide you with the net carbs used for each ½ cup serving :

- Sprouted Alfalfa Seeds (0.2)

- Arugula (2.05)

- Asparagus - 6 spears (2.4)

- Hass Avocado - half of 1 (1.8)

- Green Snap Beans (3.6)

- Beet greens (0.63)

- Bell pepper (2.1)

- Broccoli (4)

- Savoy Cabbage (3)

- Carrots (6.8)

- Baby Carrots (5.3)

- Cauliflower (3)

- Celery (1.4)

- Chard (2.1)

- Chicory Greens (0.7)

- Chives (1.9)

- Coriander/Cilantro Leaves (0.9)

- Cucumber - With Peel (3.1)

- Eggplant (2.9)

- Garlic (31)

- Ginger Root (16)

- Kale (5.2)

- Leeks With Bulb + Lower Leaf 12.4)

- Lemongrass/Citronella (25)

- Red Leaf Lettuce (1.4)

- Iceberg Lettuce (1.8)

- Brown Mushrooms (3.7)

- Mustard Greens (1.5)

- Yellow Onions (7.6)

- Scallions/Spring Onions (4.7)

- Sweet Onions (6.7)

- Banana Peppers (2)

- Red Hot Chili Peppers (7.3)

- Jalapeno Peppers (3.7)

- Sweet Green Peppers (2.9)

- Sweet Red Peppers (3.93

- Sweet Yellow Peppers (5.4)

- Portabella Mushrooms (2.6)

- Pumpkin (6)

- Radishes (1.8)

- Kelp Seaweed (8.3)

- Spirulina Seaweed (2)

- Shiitake Mushrooms (4.3)

- Spinach (1.4)

- Crookneck Summer Squash (2.6)

- Winter Acorn Squash (8.9)

- Tomatoes (2.7)

- Turnips (4.6)

- Turnip Greens (3.9)

- Summer Squash (2.6)

- Raw Watercress (3.6)

- White Mushrooms (2.3)

- Zucchini (1.5)

Purchase Keto-Friendly Fresh Fruits

The following group of fruits has been tallied as net carbs - some are noted as total carbs - for ½ cup servings (100 grams):

- Boiled Apples – no skin (13.6)

- Apricots (7.5)

- Bananas (23.4)

- Fresh Blackberries (5.4)

- Fresh Blueberries (8.2)

- Fresh Strawberries (3)

- Cantaloupe (6)

- Raw Cranberries (4)

- Gooseberries (8.8)

- Kiwi (14.2)

- Fresh Boysenberries (8.8)

- Oranges (11.7)

- Peaches (11.6 total carbs)

- Pears (19.2 total carbs)

- Pineapple (11 total carbs

- Plums (16.3 total carbs

- Watermelon- 7.1 total carbs

Choose Healthy Fats:

Not all fats are unhealthy.

- ***Natural Trans Fats:***You find these in meat and dairy products from grass-fed animals.

- ***Monounsaturated Fats:*** *Avocados:* Purchase this healthy food, which has 24 grams to 30 grams of healthy fats and is also high in fiber. The avocado is very filling and satisfying.

- ***Saturated Fats:***This is found in palm or coconut oil (medium-chain triglycerides (MCTs), cream, eggs, lard, ghee, butter, and red meat.

- ***Natural Polyunsaturated Fats:***Omega-3 is found in fish oil, fish, chia, and flaxseeds. For legumes, seeds, and nuts rich in Omega-6 (but just eat in small portions). The ratio of Omega-3 compared to Omega-6 should be as close as possible to 1:1.

Benefits of Ingredients Used

Apple Cider Vinegar:Who would believe the benefits you can receive from just one to two tablespoons of vinegar in an 8-ounce glass of water would help the process? You can choose the straight-up method and skip the water. These are just a few ways this helps your progress:
- Reduces cholesterol
- Excellent for detoxification

- Helps you to drop the pounds
- Improves your digestion tract
- Helps with sore muscles
- Controls sugar intake/aids in diabetes
- Strengthens your immune system
- A good energy booster
- Balances your inner body system and functions

Extra-Virgin Olive Oil (EVOO):Olive oil is one of the oldest edible oils in existence, with culinary uses dating back to at least 1000 B.C. and even more in the distance was the oil used for anointing priests and kings. It's versatile, delicious, and good for your health. Research shows that olive oil helps to prevent cardiovascular disease by protecting the integrity of your vascular system and lowering LDL - the 'bad' cholesterol. Furthermore, after new research, extra-virgin olive oil also improves the gut microbiome by increasing the growth of probiotic "Bifidobacteria" strains.

Monounsaturated fats, like the ones in olive oil, are also linked with better blood sugar regulation, including lower fasting glucose, as well as reducing inflammation throughout the body. Research further indicates extra-virgin olive oil resists oxidation during heating better than many other cooking oils. EVOO has a smoke point as high as 410° Fahrenheit. That's higher than most cooking applications call for and makes olive oil more heat stable than many other cooking fats.

Incorporate Coconut Oil:The oil is also used as one of the best ways to improve ketone levels in people with nervous system disorders, such as those with Alzheimer's. Coconut oil contains MCTs which speed up the ketosis process. Unlike many other fats, the MCTs are absorbed rapidly and go directly to the liver, where they are used for immediate energy – resulting in conversion to ketones.

The oil contains four types of these fats, 50% of which

comes from the lauric acid. Research has indicated a higher percentage may produce sustained ketosis levels because it is metabolized more gradually than other MCTs. Add coconut oil slowly to your diet because it can cause some stomach cramping or diarrhea until you adjust. Begin with one teaspoon daily, and work it up to two to three tablespoons for about one week.

Fermented Foods:Use items while on the keto plan such as coconut milk kefir, coconut milk, yogurt, pickles, sauerkraut, and kimchi to help with any digestive issues.

Peanut Butter:Purchase natural peanut butter but use caution because they do contain high counts of carbohydrates and Omega-6s. Macadamia nut butter is a wise alternative.

Pastured Pork & Poultry: Choose from duck, pheasant, or quail, turkey breasts & ground turkey. Enjoy chicken thighs, breasts, drumsticks, and ground chicken.

Fish:It's preferable to eat any fish that are caught in the wild. Include one single can of sardines (4 ounces) to receive 1,363 mg of omega-3 fatty acids, and nearly 400 IU of vitamin D. Raw shrimp is 5 grams of net carbs for ¼ pound. Imitation crab is 4.6 grams of net carbs for one ounce. Squid is nine grams for ¼ pound. You can also include fresh or canned tuna, trout, salmon, eel, catfish, flounder, cod, halibut, mahi-mahi, snapper, or mackerel as part of your diet plan. Just portion into bags and freeze until needed.

It is suggested by the dietary guidelines for Americans to consume at least eight ounces of fish per week. It contains an abundance of Vitamin D as well as healthy fat and protein. Fish and seafood are also good for your brain and will help with cognition and clarity while limiting the number of calories you're consuming.

Shellfish: Choose crabs, clams, lobster, oysters, scallops, squid, shrimp, or mussels.

Meat:Grass-fed meats are preferred because they have a better fatty acid count. Choose from veal, lamb, goat, or other wild game. Cuts of beef include chuck roast, flank steak, sirloin, or lean ground beef.

Venison: This is an excellent choice since it is lean, and is grass-raised meat.

Fresh Nuts: Nuts have more minerals than many other foods. Brazil nuts can be added to your diet daily as they are very high in selenium, which is vital for your immune system. It also assists your thyroid function. Walnuts are another great source of omega-3 fatty acids, protein, and fiber. The combo will fill you up and prevent blood sugar spikes. Almonds, hazelnuts, macadamia, pecans, pine nuts, cashews, or pistachios are also good choices.

Fresh Seeds*:* Pumpkin seeds are an excellent source of magnesium to include in your keto plan. They help immensely with your blood sugar levels and muscles. Flax seeds also provide an offering of omega-3 fatty acids. The micronutrients found in flax help reduce inflammation in your body. Sesame seeds, chia seeds, or psyllium are also good options. Coconut is also a good choice that can be used as shredded and unsweetened, which weighs in at .25 cup for just 1.3 net carbs.

Garlic:Garlic leads the charge on lowering your blood sugar and assisting you in weight loss. It helps control your appetite.

Lemon and Lime: Your blood sugar levels will naturally drop with these citric additions, and signal a boost in your liver function. Use them in green juices, with a salad, or with cooked meat or veggies. The choices are limitless and assist you with the following:

- Reduces toothache pain
- Boosts your immune system
- Relieves respiratory infections
- Balances pH
- Decreases wrinkles and blemishes
- Reduces fever
- Excellent for weight loss
- Flushes out the unwanted, unhealthy materials
- Blood purifier

Choose Healthy Sweeteners

Consider each one of these sweeteners before you make a choice. The recipes are usually flexible, but many typically recommend using a specific product.

Swerve Granular Sweetener is also an excellent option as a blend made from non-digestible carbs sourced from starchy root veggies and select fruits. It is an excellent choice for those who do not like the taste of stevia.

Swerve is on the market as a one-to-one substitute. However, start with ¾ of a teaspoon for every one of sugar. Increase the portion as needed. Swerve also has its own confectioners/powdered sugar for your baking needs. On the downside, it is more expensive than other products such as the Pyure.

Stevia Drops offer flavors, including English toffee, hazelnut, vanilla, and chocolate. You can make sweetened coffee or drinks quickly. However, everyone is different, and some think the drops are too bitter to taste. Therefore, only use three drops to equal one teaspoon of sugar.

Pyure Organic All-Purpose Blend is an excellent all-around sweetener. There's no bitter aftertaste with this stevia-based product. The blend of stevia and erythritol is an excellent alternative to your sweetening, baking, and cooking needs. It is suggested that you substitute 1/3 teaspoon of Pyure for every one teaspoon of sugar. Adjust this to your taste, since you can always add a bit more.

For powdered sugar, you can grind the sweetener in a NutriBullet or other blender until it's very dry.

The Purist is provided by NOW Foods has a 100% erythritol sweetener. The product is about 70% sweet as sugar. Therefore, you need a little more. Start by using 1.33 to 1.5 teaspoons of the erythritol in comparison to one teaspoon of sugar.

Lakanto provides an apple-flavored - sugar-free syrup with a monk-fruit and erythritol based. You can also select the *Golden Monk Fruit Sweetener* as a brown sugar choice. The name monk-fruit came from the Buddhist monks over 1,000 years ago. It is considered a cooling-agent and may not agree with your digestive system. Use it sparingly if using it in baked goods.

Sukrin Gold provides a brown sugar alternative. The mixture of stevia and erythritol claims the one-to-one ratio for sugar. It is always best to start with the rate of ¾ of a teaspoon per one teaspoon of sugar. According to the standards in the United States, this is not a good choice if you are seeking a gluten-free alternative because it contains malt extract.

Benefits of Spices Used

Black Pepper:Pepper can promote nutrient absorption in the body tissues, speeds up your metabolism for up to 8% for several hours as it improves digestion. The main ingredient of pepper is a pipeline, which gives it the pungent taste. As you will see, it is used throughout your ketogenic recipes.

Cayenne Pepper:The secret fiery ingredient in cayenne is the capsaicin, which is a natural compound that provides a slight increase in your metabolism. The peppers are also rich in vitamins, which are useful as an appetite controller, smooths out digestion issues, and benefit your heart health.

Cinnamon: Use cinnamon as part of your daily plan to improve your insulin receptor activity. Just put one-half of a teaspoon of cinnamon into a shake or any type of keto dessert. As you will see, many of the keto recipes contain the ingredient.

Ginger Benefits: Ginger is an effective diuretic that increases urine elimination. It is also known for its cholesterol-fighting properties, as a metabolism booster, and is even considered a mobility booster. Ginger also helps fight bloating issues, especially for women who experience weight gain and bloating during those times of the month.

Turmeric:The use of this Asian orange herb dates back to Ayurveda and Chinese medicine. The curcumin, which is an anti-inflammatory compound found in turmeric, helps improve your insulin receptor function while regulating your blood sugar levels. It aids in digestion and improves weight management. Add turmeric to your meats, vegetables, green drinks, or smoothies. To maximize the antioxidant elements, add the turmeric after the meal has finished cooking.

Mustard Seed:Spicy mustard can help boost your metabolism and allow you to burn fat quickly. This is, in fact, due to its thermogenic properties. Try substituting mayonnaise with mustard. They have the same creamy texture, and you'll only be spending about one-tenth of the calories.

Find us on Instagram, where we share contents and photos
about the book and the Ketogenic world:

easy.everydayketo
Andrew Shelby
https://www.instagram.com/easy.everydayketo

Chapter 2: Delicious Breakfast & Brunch Specialties

Bacon & Brie Frittata

Servings Provided:6
Macro Counts - Per Serving:
- Net Carbs: 1.7 g
- Calories: 338
- Protein: 18 g
- Fat Content: 27 g

Ingredients:
- Slices of bacon (8)
- Eggs (8 large)
- Heavy whipping cream (.5 cup)
- Garlic (2 cloves)
- Salt and black pepper (.5 tsp. each)
- Brie sliced thin (easiest to do when it's cold (4 oz.)
- Also Needed: 10-inch oven-proof skillet

Preparation Technique:

1. Chop and fry the bacon in the skillet using the medium heat temperature setting until it is crispy. Transfer it to drain on a paper towel-lined plate. (Leave at least 2-3 tbsp. of bacon grease in the skillet and remove from heat). Let the skillet cool.
2. Mince the garlic. Whisk the eggs with the garlic, salt, pepper, cream, and about ⅔ of the cooked bacon. Set the skillet over medium-low heat and swirl the remaining bacon grease to coat its bottom and sides.
3. Add the mix to the skillet (undisturbed) and cook for seven to ten minutes, leaving it somewhat loose to add the brie and rest of the bacon.
4. Warm the broiler and place the skillet on the second-highest rack.
5. Broil for about two to five minutes. Remove the pan and cool it for a couple of minutes to serve.

Bacon & Egg Breakfast Muffins

Servings Provided: 12
Macro Counts - Per Serving:
- Calories: 69
- Net Carbs: 0.4 g
- Protein: 5.6 g
- Fat Content: 4.9 g

Ingredients:
- Bacon slices (8)
- Eggs (8 large)
- Green onion (.66 cup)

Preparation Technique:
1. Heat the oven at 350° Fahrenheit. Spritz the muffin tin slots using a cooking oil spray.
2. Prepare a skillet using the medium temperature setting. Fry the bacon until it's crispy, and place it onto a layer of paper towels to drain the grease. Chop it into small bits after it has cooled.
3. Chop the onions. Whisk the eggs, bacon, and green onions, mixing well.
4. Dump the egg mixture into the muffin tin (half full).
5. Bake it for about 20 to 25 minutes. Cool slightly and serve.

BLT Wrap For Brunch

Servings Provided: 1
Macro Counts - Per Serving:
- Calories: 256
- Net Carbs: 2 g
- Protein: 8 g
- Fat Content: 24 g

Ingredients:
- Romaine or Iceberg lettuce leaves (2)
- Crispy fried bacon slices (4)
- Chopped tomatoes (.25 cup)
- Mayo (1 tbsp.)
- Optional: Pepper

Preparation Technique:
1. Rinse the leaves of lettuce and let them drain in a colander.
2. Prepare the bacon in a skillet or the microwave until it's crispy.
3. Spread a layer of mayonnaise on one side of the lettuce.
4. Chop and add the tomatoes and bacon bits. Season the wrap as desired.
5. Roll it up and serve.

Breakfast Skillet

Servings Provided:2
Macro Counts - Per Serving:
- Calories: 556
- Net Carbs: 7.1 g
- Protein: 65.2 g
- Fat Content: 32 g

Ingredients:
- Organic ground turkey/grass-fed beef (.75-1 lb.)
- Organic eggs (6)
- Keto-friendly salsa of choice (1 cup)

Preparation Technique:
1. Warm the skillet and add the oil (medium heat). Add the turkey/beef and simmer until the pink is gone.
2. Fold in the salsa and simmer for two to three minutes.
3. Crack the eggs and add them to the top of the turkey base. Place a lid on the pot and cook for seven minutes until the whites of the eggs are opaque.
4. *Note*: The cooking time will vary depending on how you like the eggs prepared.

Eggs Benedict Quiche

Servings Provided:8
Macro Counts - Per Serving:
- Net Carbs: 3.8 g
- Calories: 361
- Protein: 18.1 g
- Fat Content: 28.9 g

Ingredients:
The Quiche:
- Press-in pie crust (see recipe - dessert section)
- Canadian bacon (8 oz.)
- Eggs (6 large)
- Heavy whipping cream (.5 cup)
- Cloves garlic (2)
- Salt (1 tsp.)
- Pepper (.5 tsp.)
The Hollandaise:
- Eggs (2 yolks)
- Lemon juice (2 tsp.)
- Salt (.25 tsp.)
- Melted unsalted butter melted (.25 cup)
- Cayenne pepper (.125 tsp.)
- Chopped parsley for garnish
- Also Needed: Ceramic or glass container

Preparation Technique
1. Prepare the crust and warm the oven to reach 325° Fahrenheit.
2. Chop/mince the bacon and garlic. Melt the butter.
3. Press the crust into a pie dish and bake it for 12 minutes.
4. Transfer it to the countertop to add the bacon.
5. Whisk the pepper, garlic, salt, cream, and eggs. Bake for 30-40 minutes. The center should still have a little jiggle. Let it cool.

6. Prepare the hollandaise by blending the salt, juice, and yolks in a blender using the high setting for about 15 seconds.
7. With the blender running, remove the blender lid insert and place a small funnel with a narrow stem into the hole.
8. Pour in the melted butter and cayenne. Drizzle over the quiche and top it with chopped parsley as desired.

Green Buttered Eggs

Servings Provided:2
Macro Counts - Per Serving:
- Calories: 311
- Net Carbs: 2.5 g
- Protein: 13 g
- Fat Content: 27.5 g

Ingredients:
- Cloves of garlic (2)
- Fresh cilantro (.5 cup)
- Fresh parsley (.5 cup)
- Fresh thyme leaves (1 tsp.)
- Coconut oil (1 tbsp.)
- Organic butter (2 tbsp.)
- Organic eggs (4)
- Ground cayenne (.25 tsp.)
- Sea salt (.25 tsp.)
- Ground cumin (.25 tsp.)

Preparation Technique:
1. Finely chop the parsley and cilantro. Mince the garlic.
2. Warm a skillet to melt the oil and butter. Toss in the garlic and sauté it for three minutes (low setting). Sprinkle it using the thyme. Sauté for another 30 seconds.
3. Toss in the cilantro and parsley to cook using the medium heat temperature setting for about three more minutes.
4. Break in the eggs (don't break the yolk).
5. Cover the pot and cook it for 4-6 minutes or until the yolks are set (runny yolk is 3-4 minutes).
6. Serve immediately.

Mini Bacon & Kale Frittatas

Servings Provided:2
Macro Counts - Per Serving:
- Net Carbs: 4.07 g
- Calories: 285
- Protein: 16.53 g
- Fat Content: 20.69 g

Ingredients:
- Eggs (3 large)
- Whipping cream (3 tbsp.)
- Black pepper and salt (.25 tsp. each)
- Garlic powder (.125 tsp.)
- Optional: Red pepper flakes (as desired)
- Sliced bacon (4)
- Kale leaves (2 oz. - chopped)
- Also Needed: Ramekins (2 - 1 cup each)

Preparation Technique:
1. Warm the oven at 350° Fahrenheit.
2. Cover the ramekins.
3. Whisk together cream, salt, pepper, eggs, garlic powder, and pepper flakes. Set aside.
4. Prepare a medium skillet to cook bacon using medium heat until it's crispy. Drain it on a paper-lined platter and reserve two tablespoons of the bacon fat. Add the kale to the skillet to sauté until it's just tender.
5. Divide the kale between the ramekins and sprinkle with crumbled bacon. Divide the egg mixture between the ramekins.
6. Bake it for 12-15 minutes, until the frittatas are puffed and fully set.
7. Remove and serve in ramekins or let cool a few minutes and flip it out onto plates.

Mushroom Spinach Frittata

Servings Provided:6
Macro Counts - Per Serving:
- Net Carbs: 1 g
- Calories: 235
- Protein: 12 g
- Fat Content: 19 g

Ingredients:
- Avocado oil (4 tbsp. - divided)
- Cremini mushrooms (12 oz.)
- Baby spinach (2 cups - packed)
- Eggs (6 large)
- Shredded cheese blend (Monterey jack, mozzarella, cheddar (.75 cup - divided)
- Salt & pepper (1 pinch)

Preparation Technique:
1. Set the oven at 400º Fahrenheit.
2. Prepare an oven-safe skillet using the med-high temperature setting, and warm three tablespoons of oil.
3. Slice and add the mushrooms to sauté until almost tender. Toss in the spinach and sauté one minute. Remove them and lower the temperature to medium.
4. Whisk the eggs, pepper, salt, and ½ cup of cheese.
5. Pour one tablespoon of oil into the pan to cover all sides and bottom.
6. Add the egg mix, mushrooms, and spinach. Simmer for 3-4 minutes until the sides start to set.
7. Top with the remainder of the cheese. Bake it for 4-5 minutes or until the middle is almost set. Then, broil it on high for two minutes until the top is browned as desired.
8. Transfer the frittata on the countertop to cool for 5-10 minutes before slicing and serving.

9. Sprinkle it using freshly chopped parsley and salt or pepper as desired.

Pigs in Pancakes

Servings Provided:10 pancakes
Macro Counts - Per Serving:
- Net Carbs: 3.04 g
- Calories: 213
- Protein: 12.72 g
- Fat Content: 16.23 g

Ingredients:
- Almond flour - super-fine (1 cup)
- Coconut flour (.25 cup)
- Swerve sweetener (3 tbsp.)
- Salt (.25 tsp.)
- Baking powder (2 tsp.)
- Large eggs (4)
- Almond milk - unsweetened (.66 cup)
- Avocado oil/butter/ghee (.25 cup - melted)
- Vanilla extract (.5 tsp.)
- Butter or oil for a pan
- Breakfast sausages (10)
- For the Pan: Oil or butter as needed

Preparation Technique:
1. First, cook and cool the sausage.
2. Warm the oven to reach 300° Fahrenheit. Prepare a cookie sheet with a baking rack inside.
3. Whisk both types of flour with the swerve, salt, and baking powder. Whisk and add in the eggs, melted butter, milk, and vanilla extract until it's thoroughly combined.
4. Warm a skillet with butter using the medium temperature setting.
5. Use about two tablespoons of batter to create a thin line as long as your breakfast sausages (it will spread a bit as it heats up). Place the cooked sausage in the middle and cover it with another tablespoon or so of

batter. Continue to fill the pan and cook them for two to three minutes on the first side.
6. Carefully flip it over and continue cooking for another two to three minutes. Transfer them to the prepared baking rack and bake them for 10-15 minutes.
7. Note: Bob's Red Mill provides a high-quality flour for this recipe.

Pumpkin Spice Egg Loaf

Servings Provided:2
Macro Counts - Per Serving:
- Net Carbs: 2.6 g
- Calories: 277
- Protein: 8.3 g
- Fat Content: 23.4 g

Ingredients:
- Unchilled cream cheese - softened (2 oz.)
- Eggs (2 large)
- Unchilled butter (2 tbsp. softened)
- Pure pumpkin (2 tbsp.)
- Swerve sweetener (1.5 tbsp.)
- Pumpkin pie spice (.5-1 tsp.)
- Also Needed: Ramekins (2 - 8 oz. capacity)

Preparation Technique:
1. Warm the oven to reach 350° Fahrenheit.
2. Combine all of the fixings into a blender, mixing until smooth, and add to the lightly greased ramekins.
3. Bake until they are puffy (25-30 min.). Let them cool slightly and top with the spice or your favorite low-carb maple syrup (adjusting the carbs if needed).

Roasted Tomato & Pecorino Breakfast Frittata

Servings Provided:6
Macro Counts - Per Serving:

- Net Carbs: 2.4 g
- Calories: 281
- Protein: 15.73 g
- Fat Content: 21.78 g

Ingredients:

- Tomatoes (3 medium)
- Olive oil (2 tbsp.)
- Salt and pepper (to your liking)
- Eggs (8 large)
- Whipping cream (.5 cup)
- Coarsely grated Pecorino (1.5 cups - divided)
- Garlic (2 cloves)
- Salt (.5 tsp.)
- Pepper (.25 tsp.)
- Butter (2 tbsp.)
- Also Needed: 10-inch sauté pan

Preparation Technique:

1. Warm the oven to 400° Fahrenheit.
2. Slice the tomatoes (½-inch) and layer them into a glass baking dish with a drizzle of oil, pepper, and salt.
3. Bake it until tomatoes have become lightly browned and caramelized (for 40-45 min.). Set it aside to cool.
4. Mince the garlic. Whisk the whipping cream, eggs, one cup of the grated Pecorino, salt, pepper, and garlic.
5. Melt the butter in the pan using the medium temperature setting, swirling to coat the entire pan. Dump in the egg mixture and reduce the heat setting to med-low. Cook them undisturbed for about 10

minutes. Warm the broiler to high and set a rack to the second-highest setting in the oven.

6. Lay roasted tomato slices over top of the frittata and sprinkle with the remaining pecorino.
7. Broil it until it's lightly browned (5 min.) and serve.

Sausage & Cheese Omelet Roll

Servings Provided: 6/1 roll
Macro Counts - Per Serving:

- Net Carbs: 3.45 g
- Calories: 412
- Protein: 23 g
- Fat Content: 30.9 g

Ingredients:

- Butter or avocado oil (1 tbsp.)
- Al Fresco® Country-Style chicken breakfast sausage (7- oz pkg.)
- Eggs (8 large)
- Cream cheese (4 oz.)
- Whipping cream (.5 cup)
- Salt (1 tsp.)
- Pepper (.5 tsp.)
- Garlic powder (.5 tsp.)
- Cheddar (1.5 cups - divided)
- Also Needed: 11x17 inch rimmed baking sheet

Preparation Technique:

1. Prepare a large skillet using the medium temperature setting to melt the butter. Add the sausage and cook until done, remove it from the pan, and thinly slice it.
2. Warm the oven to reach 350° Fahrenheit.
3. Prepare the baking tray with a layer of parchment paper and spritz it using a cooking oil spray.
4. Use a blender to mix the garlic powder, salt, pepper, whipping cream, cream cheese, and eggs.
5. Pour it into the pan and bake it for 15-18 minutes until it's just cooked through. Remove and sprinkle it with one cup of cheese and a sprinkle of the sausage.
6. Start at the short end and roll it. Sprinkle with the rest of the cheddar and bake five minutes before slicing to serve.

Sausage Gravy & Biscuits

Servings Provided:2
Macro Counts - Per Serving:
- Calories: 425
- Net Carbs: 2 g
- Protein: 22 g
- Fat Content: 36 g

Ingredients:

- Salt (.25 tsp.)

- Almond flour (.25 cup)

- Baking powder (.5 tsp.)

- Large egg white (1)

- Crumbled breakfast sausage (6 oz. pkg.)

- Chicken broth (.25 cup)

- Cream cheese (.25 cup)

- Pepper and salt (as desired)

Preparation Technique:
1. Warm the oven at 400° Fahrenheit. Prepare a baking tin with a sheet of parchment baking paper.
2. Whisk the salt, almond flour, and baking powder.
3. In another dish, whisk the egg whites to form stiff peaks.
4. Dice the butter into small pieces. Form a crumbled mixture in the dry components using the butter. Gently blend into the egg whites.
5. Split the mixture into two portions on the paper-lined pan.

6. Bake them for 11 to 15 minutes.
7. Using the medium heat setting to warm the sausage. When browned, add the cream cheese, chicken broth, pepper, and salt.
8. Serve with the biscuits and a serving of the delicious gravy.
9. Prep time is just 15 minutes with a cooking time of only 25 minutes. What a treat in such a little amount of time!

Southwestern Cauliflower Breakfast Pizza

Servings Provided:432
Macro Counts - Per Serving:
- Net Carbs: 2.6 g
- Calories: 9.7
- Protein: 28.3 g
- Fat Content: 28.6 g

Ingredients:
> *The Crust:*
- Riced cauliflower (12 oz./about 1 medium head)
- Shredded mozzarella (1 cup)
- Egg (1 large)
- Clove of garlic (1 minced)
- Black pepper and salt (.5 tsp.)
> *The Toppings:*
- Shredded cheddar cheese (1.5 cups)
- Breakfast sausage links (4 cooked and sliced)
- Jalapeno (1 sliced)
- Large eggs (4)
- Salt and pepper (as needed)
- Ripe California avocado (1 large - thinly sliced)
- Chopped tomato (.25 cup)
- Chopped cilantro for garnish
- Also Needed: 12-inch oven-proof skillet & large microwave-safe dish

Preparation Technique:
1. Set the oven at 400° Fahrenheit. Lightly spritz the skillet with a misting of oil.
2. Prepare and add the cauliflower into a microwave-safe dish and cover using plastic wrap. Set the timer for ten minutes and place on a tea towel-lined sieve over the sink until it's cooled to handle.

3. Twist the towel and remove the cauliflower to a mixing container with the salt, pepper, garlic, egg, and mozzarella. Mix it thoroughly.
4. Pour it into the skillet and bake for 18-22 minutes or when the center is firm with golden brown edges.
5. Sprinkle the crust with one cup of cheese, sausage, and jalapenos.
6. Break the eggs over the pizza, and add the cheese.
7. Bake it for 8-12 minutes until they're as desired. Garnish them with tomatoes and avocado or a sprinkle of cilantro.

Sweets Corner

Chocolate Loaf

Servings Provided:8
Macro Counts - Per Serving:
- Calories: 195
- Net Carbs: 2.32 g
- Protein: 5.7 g
- Fat Content: 17.8 g

Ingredients:
- Large eggs (6)
- Butter (4 oz.)
- Coconut flour (.75 cup)
- Baking powder (1 tsp.)
- Sugar substitute (personal preference)
- Unsweetened cocoa powder (.33 cup)
- Salt (1 pinch)
- Baking soda (.5 tsp.)
- Apple cider vinegar (2 tsp.)
- *Also Needed*: Parchment baking paper

Preparation Technique:
1. Heat the oven to reach 350° Fahrenheit.
2. Prepare a baking pan using a layer of parchment baking paper.
3. Whisk the eggs and stir in the melted butter.
4. Sift the dry fixings. Pour in the wet mixture and add the vinegar.
5. Stir well and pour into the pan.
6. Bake the loaf for 20 to 30 minutes.
7. Serve when tested in the center with a toothpick, and it comes out clean.

Cocoa Waffles

Servings Provided:5
Macro Counts - Per Serving:
- Calories: 289
- Net Carbs: 3.4 g
- Protein: 7 g
- Fat Content: 27 g

Ingredients:
- Separated eggs (5)
- Unsweetened cocoa (.25 cup)
- Baking powder (1 tsp.)
- Granular sweetener (3 tbsp.)
- Coconut flour (4 tbsp.)
- Melted butter (4.5 oz.)
- Milk of choice (3 tbsp.)
- Vanilla (1 tsp.)

Preparation Technique:
1. Use a whisk and prepare the egg whites to form stiff peaks.
2. In another container, whisk the sweetener, baking powder, and cocoa with the egg yolks.
3. Add the butter to the dry mixture. Stir in the vanilla and milk.
4. Fold in the prepared egg whites - a little at a time.
5. Pour the mixture in the waffle maker.
6. Cook until they are nicely browned and serve.

Peanut Butter Protein Bars

Servings Provided:12
Macro Counts - Per Serving:
- Calories: 172
- Net Carbs: 3 g
- Protein: 7 g
- Fat Content: 14 g

Ingredients:
- Almond meal (1.5 cups)
- Keto-friendly chunky peanut butter (1 cup)
- Egg whites (2)
- Almonds (.5 cup)
- Cashews (.5 cup)

Preparation Technique:
1. Heat the oven ahead of time to reach 350º Fahrenheit.
2. Spritz a baking dish lightly with coconut or olive oil.
3. Combine all of the fixings and add them to the prepared dish.
4. Bake for 15 minutes and then cut into 12 pieces once they're cool.
5. Store in the refrigerator to keep them fresh.

Sugar-Free Krispy Kreme™ Doughnuts

Servings: 8
Total Time Required: 48 Minutes
Servings Provided:12
Macro Counts - Per Serving:
- Calories: 86
- Protein: 4 g
- Net Carbs: 1.3 g
- Fat Content: 7 g

Ingredients:
- Large eggs (2)
- Full-fat cream cheese (80 grams)
- Erythritol (20 grams)
- Pure stevia powder (.5 tsp.)
- Unsalted butter (20 grams)
- Vanilla whey protein powder (30 grams)
- Fine psyllium husk powder (10 grams)
- Himalayan pink salt (1 pinch)
- Baking powder (2 tsp.)
- Apple cider vinegar - ACV (1 tbsp.)
    - *Optional Frosting :*
- Mascarpone (120 grams)
- Sukrin icing sugar (15 grams)
- Vanilla extract (2-3 drops)
- Pitaya powder for pink topping
- Maqui powder for lilac topping
- Unsweetened dark chocolate - a minimum of 85%

Preparation Technique:
1. Warm the oven to reach 300° Fahrenheit.
2. Whisk the eggs, salt, cream cheese, erythritol, and stevia (in that order).
3. Melt the butter, and cool it slightly. Whisk it into the egg mix.

4. Mix in the whey, psyllium, baking powder, and ACV. Mix thoroughly.
5. Place the mixture into the doughnut molds (8 doughnuts).
6. Bake them for 18 minutes. Turn the oven to the "*off*" setting and open the door. Wait for five minutes before taking them out.
7. Cool the doughnuts completely, and remove them from the molds.
8. Prepare the Frosting: Beat the mascarpone until soft, then incorporate the icing sugar, mixing thoroughly.
9. Choose the type of frosting and spread it over the tops.
10. Note: On average, the Krispy Kreme version is 22 carbs versus the Keto version of 1.3 net carbs.

Chapter 3: Luncheon Salad & Pasta

Salad Options

Greek Chopped Salad

Servings Provided:2
Macro Counts - Per Serving:
- Net Carbs: 2 g
- Calories: 202
- Protein: 4 g
- Fat Content: 19 g

Ingredients:
- Chopped romaine (2 cups)
- Halved grape tomatoes (.5 cup)
- Kalamata black olives (.25 cup)
- Crumbled feta cheese (.25 cup)
- Olive oil (1 tbsp.)
- Vinaigrette dressing (2 tbsp.)
- Black pepper & Pink salt (as desired)

Preparation Technique:
1. Put the salad together using the lettuce as a base.
2. Spritz it using a drizzle of oil and vinegar.
3. Serve in two salad dishes.

Greek Meatball Salad

Servings Provided:4
Macro Counts - Per Serving:
- Net Carbs: 2 g
- Calories: 399
- Protein: 20 g
- Fat Content: 36 g

Ingredients:
- Finely chopped mint (.25 cup)
- Garlic cloves (2 minced)
- Pepper and salt (to your liking)
- Dried oregano (2 tsp.)
- Ground lamb/beef (1 lb.)
- Olive oil (4 tbsp.)
    - *The Salad:*
- Lettuce leaves (2-3)
- Tomato (1)
- Lemon (1)
- Chopped flat-leaf parsley (.25 cup)

Preparation Technique:
1. Set the oven at 350° Fahrenheit. Slice the tomato and lemon into wedges.
2. Combine the spices and meat and shape into meatballs. Portion the mixture for four servings.
3. Warm the olive oil in a skillet until the meatballs are lightly browned. Arrange on a baking tin. Cook them for ten minutes.
4. Serve over the prepared salad with a garnish of lemon and parsley.

Jar Salad

Servings Provided:1
Macro Counts - Per Serving:

- Net Carbs: 4 g
- Calories: 215
- Protein: 8 g
- Fat Content: 19 g

Ingredients:

- Black pepper & salt (as desired)

- Keto-friendly mayonnaise (4 tbsp.)

- Scallion (.5)

- Cucumber (.25 oz.)

- Red bell pepper (.25 oz.)

- Cherry tomatoes (.25 oz.)

- Leafy greens (.25 oz.)

- Seasoned tempeh (4 oz.)

Preparation Technique:

1. Chop or shred the vegetables as desired. Layer in the dark leafy greens first, followed by the onions, tomato, bell peppers, avocado, and shredded carrot.
2. Top with the tempeh, or use the same amount of another high-protein option to mix things up in later weeks.
3. Top with keto mayonnaise before serving.

Kiwi & Feta Chicken Salad

Servings Provided:2
Macro Counts - Per Serving:
- Net Carbs: 13 g
- Calories: 314
- Protein: 28 g
- Fat Content: 15 g

Ingredients:
- Fig balsamic vinegar (1 tbsp.)
- Kiwi (2)
- Olive oil (1 tbsp.)
- Salt (1 pinch)
- Mixed field greens (4 cups)
- Chopped grilled chicken breast (1 cup - about 5 oz.)
- Feta cheese (.33 cup)

Preparation Technique:
1. Chop the chicken and crumble the feta.
2. Whisk the balsamic vinegar, oil, and salt.
3. Add the greens and chicken breast.
4. Peel and cut the kiwi into halves. Dice into 1-inch wedges and add to the salad with the crumbled feta.
5. Toss well to combine.

Pecan & Chicken Salad with Cucumber Bites

Servings Provided:2
Macro Counts - Per Serving:
- Net Carbs: 3 g
- Calories: 323
- Protein: 23 g
- Fat Content: 24 g

Ingredients:

- Cucumber (1)

- Precooked chicken breast (1 cup)

- Celery (.25 cup)

- Mayonnaise (2 tbsp.)

- Pecans (.25 cup)

Preparation Technique:
1. Peel and slice the cucumber into ¼-inch slices. Dice the chicken and celery. Chop the pecans.
2. Combine the pecans, chicken, mayonnaise, and celery in a salad bowl. Sprinkle with pepper and salt if desired.
3. Prepare the cucumber slices. Layer each one with a spoonful of the chicken salad. Serve any time of the day or night.

Steak Salad

Servings Provided:2
Macro Counts - Per Serving:
- Net Carbs: 1.5 g
- Calories: 403
- Protein: 1.5 g
- Fat Content: 33 g

Ingredients:
- Steakhouse seasoning (1 tbsp.)
- Pepper and salt (to taste)
- Ribeye steak (1- 8 oz.)
- Green salad mix (2 cups)
- Wine vinegar (1 tsp.)
- Olive oil (1 tbsp.)

Preparation Technique:
1. Use the steak seasoning to prepare the steak and cook as desired.
2. Wait for it to cool while you toss the salad fixings with a dusting of pepper and salt.
3. Drizzle with oil and toss again.
4. Slice the steak into bite-sized strips.
5. Arrange the salad on two serving dishes and sprinkle the steak bits on top.
6. Serve using your favorite dressing if desired - but count the carbs.

Tuna Salad & Chives

Servings Provided: 4
Macro Counts - Per Serving:
- Net Carbs: 1 g
- Calories: 235
- Protein: 20 g
- Fat Content: 18 g

Ingredients:
- Tuna - packed in olive oil (15 oz.)
- Mayonnaise (6 tbsp.)
- Chives (2 tbsp.)
- Pepper (.25 tsp.)

Preparation Technique:
1. Drain the tuna and finely chop the chives.
2. Add all of the fixings except the lettuce into a mixing bowl.
3. Toss well. Enjoy as-is or spoon into romaine lettuce leaves.

Pasta & Meatball Options

2 Ingredient Keto Pasta

Servings: 1
Nutritional Facts Per Serving:
- Net Carbs: 3 g
- Calories: 358
- Protein: 33 g
- Fat Content: 22 g

Ingredients:
- Large egg yolk (1)
- Shredded mozzarella cheese - part-skim - low moisture (1 cup/113 g)

Preparation Technique:
1. Prepare the mozzarella using a large microwave-safe bowl. Set the timer on the microwave for one minute. Stir until the cheese is melted at 30-second intervals.
2. Pop the mixture into the fridge for one minute (chill slightly), so that it will not cook the egg. Stir the egg yolk into the cheese.
3. Place the dough onto a cutting block prepared with a layer of parchment baking paper. Add another sheet on top.
4. Flatten the dough until it's about ⅛-inch thick using a rolling pin.
5. Trash the top piece of baking paper and cut the dough into ½-inch wide strips. Place the pasta in the refrigerator for at least six hours (overnight is best).
6. Prepare a pot of unsalted water. Toss in the pasta to cook about 40 seconds to one minute.
7. Remove the pasta from the pot and run it under cold water until cooled.
8. Gently separate the strands if they're sticking together. Chill until it's only slightly warm to the touch. It will become firm again after it cools. Serve alongside your favorite pasta sauce.

Creamy Salmon Pasta

Servings Provided: 2
Macro Counts - Per Serving:
- Net Carbs: 3 g
- Calories: 470
- Protein: 21 g
- Fat Content: 42 g

Ingredients:
- *Zucchinis (2)*
- *Coconut oil (2 tbsp.)*
- *Smoked salmon (8 oz.)*
- *Keto-friendly mayo (.25 cup)*

Preparation Technique:
1. *Prepare noodle-like strands from the zucchini using a spiralizer or vegetable peeler.*
2. *Heat the oil using the med-high heat setting. When hot, add the salmon to sauté for two to three minutes or until golden brown.*
3. *Stir in the noodles and sauté for 1 to 2 more minutes.*
4. Store the noodles in the fridge overnight after cooling.
5. When it's time to eat, stir in the mayo and divide the pasta between two dishes to serve.

Gluten-Free - Vegan Zucchini 'Meatballs'

Servings: 12 meatballs
Nutritional Facts Per Serving:
- Net Carbs: 1.1 g
- Calories: 71
- Protein: 1.7 g
- Fat Content: 6.6 g

Ingredients:
- Chopped/ground walnuts (1 cup)
- Shredded zucchini (1 cup)
- Salt (.25 tsp.)
- Dried oregano (1 tbsp.)
- Granulated garlic (.25 tsp.)
- Italian seasoning (1 tbsp.)
- Red pepper flakes (.25 tsp.)
- Psyllium husks (1 tbsp.)

Preparation Technique:
1. Set the oven temperature in advance to reach 350°Fahrenheit. Cover a baking tray using a sheet of parchment paper.
2. Mix the shredded zucchini, chopped walnuts, and salt. Wait for about five minutes for some of the moisture to be pulled from the zucchini.
3. Stir in the psyllium and seasoning until it's thoroughly combined. Wait for another five minutes for the psyllium to bind.
4. Shape the mixture into balls and place them onto the baking pan.
5. Bake until the zucchini balls are slightly browned and firm to the touch (30-35 minutes).
6. Serve over zucchini or other types of keto-friendly noodles with a low-carb red sauce, and serve.

Italian Parmesan Chicken Meatballs

Servings Provided:4
Macro Counts - Per Serving:
- Net Carbs: 3 g
- Calories: 257
- Protein: 26 g
- Fat Content: 15 g

Ingredients:
- Ground chicken (1 lb.)
- Minced garlic (3 cloves)
- Grated parmesan cheese (.25 cup)
- Freshly chopped flat-leaf parsley (3 tbsp.)
- Onion powder (.5 tsp.)
- Dried Italian seasoning (.5 tsp.)
- Black pepper (.25 tsp.)
- Sea salt (.5 tsp.)
- Shredded mozzarella cheese (.5 cup)
- Three Cheese Garlic Marinara Sauce (.5 cup)

Preparation Technique:
1. Set the oven to reach 350° Fahrenheit
2. Lightly grease a large baking dish.
3. In a large mixing container, combine two tablespoons of the marinara sauce, the ground chicken, parsley, onion powder, garlic, parmesan cheese, salt, pepper, and Italian seasoning.
4. Shape the mixture into twelve meatballs.
5. Arrange the prepared meatballs in the baking dish. Leave a small space between each meatball.
6. Bake it on the center rack of the oven for 25 minutes.
7. Once it's browned, pull it out of the oven and dump the remainder of the sauce over the top of the balls. Cover the meatballs with mozzarella cheese.
8. Set the oven temperature setting to broil.

9. Once it is hot, put the pan of meatballs on the rack to
    bake until it's golden brown for approximately two to
    three minutes.

Keto Spaghetti Sauce

Servings:16
Nutritional Facts Per Serving:
- Net Carbs: 2 g
- Calories: 249
- Protein: 16 g
- Fat Content: 17 g

Ingredients:
- Garlic cloves (6)
- Salt (1 tsp.)
- Beef stock (4 cups)
- Fat/grease (2 oz.)
- Brown onions (2 medium)
- Ground beef (3 lb.)
- Pepper (1 tsp.)
- Tomato puree (24 oz.)
- Oregano (2 tbsp.)
- Dried marjoram (1 tbsp.)
- Basil (2 tbsp.)
- Parsley (1 tbsp.)

Preparation Technique:
1. Heat the stock in a saucepan using the medium to a high-temperature setting until it's reduced to one cup of juices.
2. Melt the grease into another pan using the high-temperature setting.
3. Dice and add in the garlic, onion, marjoram, and salt. Sauté for about five minutes.
4. Fold in the beef and continue sautéing until it's browncd.
5. Reduce the temperature to add the beef stock and tomato puree.
6. Leave the lid off of the pan and cook for 1 hour to 1.25 hours. Add the rest of the fixings when it's thickened.
7. Chop the fresh parsley, oregano, and basil. Add other seasonings as desired before serving.

Zoodles & White Clam Sauce

Servings Provided:4
Macro Counts - Per Serving:
- Net Carbs: 7 g
- Calories: 311
- Protein: 13 g
- Fat Content: 19 g

Ingredients:
- Olive oil (2 tbsp.)
- Butter (.25 cup)
- Kosher salt (1 tsp.)
- Black pepper (.25 tsp.)
- Garlic (1 tbsp.)
- Dry white wine (.5 cup)
- Lemon juice (2 tbsp.)
- Baby clams (1 large can) drained or Small clams (2 lb.)
- Zucchini noodles (8 cups)
- Freshly chopped parsley (.25 cup)
- Grated lemon zest (1 tsp.)

Preparation Technique:
1. Prepare a skillet on the stovetop using the med-high temperature setting to warm the butter, oil, pepper, and salt. Mince and toss in the garlic when it's hot, and sauté for about two minutes until it's fragrant.
2. Whisk in the lemon juice and wine to sauté for two minutes.
3. Mix in the clams and continue cooking for another two to three minutes. If using canned clams, cook for two minutes. (The ones that didn't open should be discarded.)
4. Transfer to the countertop and add the noodles. Toss to cover and marinate for two minutes.
5. Stir in the lemon zest, pepper flakes, and parsley or other seasonings as desired.

Chapter 4: Lunchtime & Dinner Soups

Asiago Tomato Soup

Servings Provided:4
Macro Counts - Per Serving:
- Net Carbs: 8.75 g
- Calories: 302
- Protein: 9 g
- Fat Content: 26 g

Ingredients:
- Tomato paste (1 small can)
- Minced garlic (1 tsp.)
- Oregano (1 tsp.)
- Heavy whipping cream (1 cup)
- Water (.25 cup)
- Pepper and salt (as desired)
- Asiago cheese (.75 cup)

Preparation Technique:
1. Pour the minced garlic and tomato paste in a dutch oven and add the cream. Gently whisk.
2. As it begins to boil, blend in small amounts of cheese. Pour in the water and simmer for four to five minutes.
3. Serve with pepper as desired.

Broccoli "N" Cheese Soup - Crock Pot

Servings Provided:3
Macro Counts - Per Serving:
- Net Carbs: 6.6 g
- Calories: 215
- Protein: 3.5 g
- Fat Content: 21.4 g

Ingredients:
- Vegetable broth (1 cup)
- Broccoli (1 cup)
- Cheddar cheese (1 cup)
- Coconut cream (.5 cup)

Preparation Technique:
1. Add each of the ingredients into a crockpot.
2. Set the timer for four hours using the low setting.
3. Serve it piping hot.

Cabbage Roll 'Unstuffed' Soup

Servings Provided:9
Macro Counts - Per Serving:
- Net Carbs: 3 g
- Calories: 217
- Protein: 16 g
- Fat Content: 15 g

Ingredients:

- Minced garlic cloves (2)

- Small diced onion (.5 of 1)

- 80/20 Ground beef (1.5 lb.)

- Bragg's Aminos (.25 cup)

- Tomato sauce (8 oz. can)

- Beef broth (3 cups)

- Keto-friendly Worcestershire sauce/another substitute (3 tsp.)

- Diced tomatoes (14 oz. can)

- Chopped cabbage (1 medium)

- Pepper (.5 tsp.)

- Parsley (.5 tsp.)

- Salt (.5 tsp.)

- *Also Needed:* Instant Pot

Preparation Technique:
1. Prepare using the sauté function on the Instant Pot to

brown the beef, garlic, and onions.

2. Drain and add back to the pot with the rest of the fixings.
3. Program the unit on the soup function.
4. Natural-release the soup for about ten minutes, and quick-release the rest of the steam. Stir and serve.

Carrot - Chili Soup

Servings Provided:6
Macro Counts - Per Serving:
- Net Carbs: 3 g
- Calories: 440
- Protein: 21 g
- Fat Content: 37 g

Ingredients:
- Avocado oil (2 tbsp.)
- Ground beef (1.5 lb.)
- Cooked diced bacon (4 slices)
- Diced onion (half of 1)
- Diced tomatoes (2)
- Water (.25 cup)
- Shredded carrots (2)
- Garlic cloves (2 minced)
- Chopped cilantro (.25 cup)
- Pepper and salt (to taste)

Preparation Technique:
1. Pour the oil into a pot on the stovetop. Brown the bacon and beef using the high-temperature setting. Toss in the onion for a few minutes until browned.
2. Pour in the tomatoes, water, and carrots with some salt to your liking.
3. Simmer for about one hour (lid on), stirring often.
4. Stir in the prepared garlic and cilantro to simmer for five more minutes.
5. Taste test the soup and serve.

Chicken 'Zoodle' Soup

Servings Provided:2
Macro Counts - Per Serving:
- Net Carbs: 4 g
- Calories: 310
- Protein: 34 g
- Fat Content: 16 g

Ingredients:

- Chicken broth (3 cups)

- Chicken breast (1)

- Avocado oil (2 tbsp.)

- Green onion (1)

- Celery stalk (1)

- Cilantro (.25 cup)

- Salt (to taste)

- Peeled zucchini (1)

Preparation Technique:
1. Chop or dice the breast of the chicken. Pour the oil into a saucepan and cook the chicken until done. Pour in the broth and simmer. Chop the celery and green onions and toss into the pan. Simmer for 3 to 4 more minutes.
2. Chop the cilantro and prepare the zucchini noodles. Use a spiralizer or potato peeler to make the 'noodles.' Add to the pot.
3. Simmer for a few more minutes and season to your liking.

4. Store the leftovers in a glass container in the fridge for
    two to three days.

Chili Delight - No-Beans

Servings Provided:6
Macro Counts - Per Serving:
- Net Carbs: 5 g
- Calories: 263
- Protein: 26 g
- Fat Content: 14 g

Ingredients:
- Water (3 cups)
- Ground beef 1.5 lb.)
- Cumin (.75 tsp.)
- Black pepper (.75 tsp.)
- Cinnamon (.25 tsp.)
- Minced garlic cloves (2)
- Chopped onion (.25 cup)
- Worcestershire sauce (1 tsp.)
- Bay leaves (3)
- Chili powder (2 tbsp.)
- Salt (1.5 tsp.)
- Allspice (.5 tsp.)
- Red pepper (.5 tsp.)
- Tomato paste (6 oz.)
- Sliced black olives (2.25 oz.)
- Finely chopped chili peppers (.25 cup)

Preparation Technique:
1. Break apart the ground beef in a large stew pot on the stovetop. Drain away the juices.
2. Combine with the rest of the fixings. Bring to a boil.
3. Simmer the chili for two hours and serve.

Chilled Avocado Mint Soup

Servings Provided:2
Macro Counts - Per Serving:
- Net Carbs: 4 g
- Calories: 280
- Protein: 4 g
- Fat Content: 26 g

Ingredients:
- Romaine lettuce (2 leaves)
- Ripened avocado (1 medium)
- Coconut milk (1 cup)
- Lime juice (1 tbsp.)
- Fresh mint (20 leaves)
- Salt (to your liking)

Preparation Technique:
1. Combine all of the fixings into a blender and mix well. You want it thick but not puree-like.
2. Chill in the refrigerator for five to ten minutes before serving.

Creamy Chicken Soup

Servings Provided: 4
Macro Counts - Per Serving:
- Net Carbs: 2 g
- Calories: 307
- Protein: 18 g
- Fat Content: 25 g

Ingredients:

- Butter (2 tbsp.)

- Large breast of chicken (1-2 cups - shredded)

- Cubed cream cheese (4 oz.)

- Garlic seasoning (2 tbsp.)

- Chicken broth (14.5 oz.)

- Salt (to taste)

- Heavy cream (.25 cup)

Preparation Technique:
1. Heat a saucepan and melt the butter using the medium temperature setting.
2. Mix in the shredded chicken and toss with the cream cheese and seasoning.
3. When it is all melted, stir in the heavy cream and broth.
4. Once it's boiling, lower the heat and cook slowly for three to four minutes.
5. Season the soup as desired before serving.

Curried-Style Fish Stew

Servings Provided:6
Macro Counts - Per Serving:
- Net Carbs: 8 g
- Calories: 373
- Protein: 33 g
- Fat Content: 21 g

Ingredients:
- Chopped onion (1 medium)
- Cauliflower (1 head - chopped)
- Olive oil (1 tbsp.)
- Tomato paste (1 tbsp.)
- Minced garlic (3 cloves)
- Curry powder (2 tbsp.)
- Fish/vegetable broth (2 cups)
- Firm - cubed whitefish – ex. halibut/cod (1.5 lb.)
- Ground cayenne pepper (1 tsp.)
- Black pepper and salt (to your liking)
- Full-fat coconut milk (13.5 oz. can)

Preparation Technique:
1. Heat the oil in a large saucepan using the medium temperature setting.
2. Mince and sauté the garlic and onion for 5 to 7 minutes. Once they're translucent, stir in the cauliflower, curry powder, and tomato paste. Continue sautéing for 10 to 15 minutes.
3. Sprinkle it with the salt, pepper, and cayenne. Simmer for one to two minutes more.
4. Pour in the coconut milk and simmer on low until ready to serve.
5. Store in the fridge for up to four days.

Egg Drop Soup

Servings Provided:6
Macro Counts - Per Serving:
- Net Carbs: 3 g
- Calories: 255
- Protein: 11 g
- Fat Content: 22 g

Ingredients:
- Vegetable broth (2 quarts)
- Freshly chopped ginger (1 tbsp.)
- Turmeric (1 tbsp.)
- Sliced chili pepper (1 small)
- Coconut aminos (2 tbsp.)
- Minced garlic cloves (2)
- Large eggs (4)
- Mushrooms (2 cups)
- Chopped spinach (4 cups)
- Sliced spring onions (2 medium)
- Freshly chopped cilantro (2 tbsp.)
- Black pepper (to your liking)
- Pink Himalayan (1 tsp.)
- For serving: Olive oil (6 tbsp.)

Preparation Technique:
1. Prep the Fixings: Grate the ginger root and turmeric. Mince the garlic cloves and slice the peppers and mushrooms.
2. Chop the chard stalks and leaves. Separate the stalks from the leaves. Dump the vegetable stock into a soup pot and simmer until it begins to boil. Toss in the garlic, ginger, turmeric, chard stalks, mushrooms, coconut aminos, and chili peppers. Boil for approximately five minutes.
3. Fold in the chard leaves and simmer for one minute.
4. Whip the eggs in a dish and add them slowly to the soup mixture. Stir until the egg is done and set it on

the counter.

5. Slice the onions and chop the cilantro. Toss them into the pot.
6. Pour into serving bowls and drizzle with some olive oil (1 tbsp. per serving).

Healthy Green Soup

Servings Provided:6
Macro Counts - Per Serving:
- Net Carbs: 6 g
- Calories: 191
- Protein: 6 g
- Fat Content: 8 g

Ingredients:
- Spinach leaves (2 cups)
- Diced avocado (1)
- Diced English cucumber (.5 cup)
- Gluten-free vegetable broth (.25 cup)
- Black pepper and salt (as desired)

Preparation Technique:
1. Toss the ingredients into a blender.
2. Add the fresh herbs and serve it.

Sausage Kale & Mushroom Soup

Servings Provided:6
Macro Counts - Per Serving:
- Net Carbs: 4 g
- Calories: 259
- Protein: 14 g
- Fat Content: 20 g

Ingredients:
- Fresh kale (6.5 oz.)
- Sausage (1 lb.)
- Mushrooms (6.5 oz.)
- Garlic (2 cloves)
- Chicken bone broth (29 oz.)

Preparation Technique:
1. Slice the mushrooms and mince the garlic. Chop the kale into bite-sized pieces. Remove the casings and cook the sausage.
2. Pour in the broth with two cans of water. Boil using the medium temperature setting.
3. Toss in the rest of the fixings using the low-heat setting and simmer for one hour.

Chapter 5: Sandwiches - Snacks & Appetizers

Sandwiches

Philly Cheesesteak

Servings Provided:1
Macro Counts - Per Serving:
- Net Carbohydrates: 6 g
- Calories: 461
- Protein: 21 g
- Fat Content: 38 g

Ingredients:
- Green pepper (half of 1)
- Onion (.25 cup)
- Oil or butter (as needed)
- Steak (1)
- Mushrooms (1 oz. canned)
- Pepper and salt (as desired)
- Mozzarella or provolone cheese (.5 oz.)

Preparation Technique:
1. Slice or chop the peppers and onions. Drain the can of mushrooms (4 oz. size - ¼ of the can).
2. Season the steak to your liking and chop into bite-sized pieces or leave it whole.
3. Sauté it in a skillet with the oil, onions, mushrooms, and green peppers.
4. Top off the steak with the veggies and a layer of cheese.
5. Heat the oven and broil the sandwich for a minute or so to melt the cheese.

Shrimp & Fish Roe Salad Sandwiches

Servings Provided:4
Macro Counts - Per Serving:
- Net Carbs: 2 g
- Calories: 496
- Protein: 14 g
- Fat Content: 48 g

Ingredients:
- Shrimp (10 oz.)
- Mayonnaise (1 cup)
- Sour cream/crème fraîche (.25 cup)
- Fresh dill (2 tbsp.)
- Fish roe (2 oz.)
- Lemon juice (2 tsp.)
- Salt and pepper (as desired)

Preparation Technique:
1. Peel, cook, and roughly chop half of the shrimp.
2. Whisk the mayo and sour cream in a mixing container.
3. Fold in the dill, roe, and shrimp. Reserve a portion for garnishing.
4. Dust the sandwich salad using the pepper and salt and a drizzle of lemon juice before serving.

Other Snacks & Appetizers

Air-Fried Taco Meatballs

Servings Provided:4
Macro Counts - Per Serving:
- Net Carbs: 5 g
- Calories: 323
- Protein: 33 g
- Fat Content: 18 g

Ingredients:
- Lean ground beef (1 lb.)
- Onions (.25 cup)
- Cilantro (.25 cup)
- Garlic (1 tbsp.)
- Taco seasoning (2 tbsp.)
- Mexican blend shredded cheese (.5 cup)
- Eggs (1)
- Black pepper and kosher salt (as desired)
- *The Sauce:*
- Sour cream (.25 cup)
- Salsa (.5 cup)
- Hot sauce (1-2 tsp.)
- Also Needed: Stand mixer with a paddle attachment.

Preparation Technique:
1. Warm the Air Fryer at 400° Fahrenheit.
2. Dice or mince the garlic, onions, and cilantro. Add the attachment to the mixer.
3. Toss each of the fixings in the mixing bowl and blend them for about two to three minutes.
4. Shape it into 12 meatballs.
5. Place them in the basket of the Air Fryer. Set the timer for ten minutes.
6. Combine the sauce fixings and serve it with the meatballs.

Avocado - Tuna Melt Bites

Servings Provided:12
Macro Counts - Per Serving:
- Net Carbohydrates: 1 g
- Calories: 185
- Protein: 5 g
- Fat Content: 17.8 g

Ingredients:
- Mayonnaise (.25 cup)
- Parmesan cheese (.25 cup)
- Drained tuna (10 oz.)
- Almond flour (.33 cup)
- Onion powder (.25 tsp.)
- Garlic powder (.5 tsp.)
- Pepper and salt (as desired)
- Cubed avocado (1 medium)
- Coconut oil for cooking (2 tbsp.)

Preparation Technique:
1. Prepare the avocado by removing the pit. Cut it into cubes.
2. Combine each of the fixings (omitting the oil and avocado).
3. Fold in the tuna with the avocado and shape into balls. Coat with flour.
4. Heat the oil using the medium temperature setting and fry until browned. Serve or store when it's cooled.

Beef Satay

Servings Provided:2
Macro Counts - Per Serving:
- Net Carbs: 0.7 g
- Calories: 328
- Protein: 43.4 g
- Fat Content: 15.8 g

Ingredients:
- Beef brisket (10 oz.)
- Chili paste (.5 tsp.)
- Coconut oil (1 tbsp.)
- Stevia (1 tsp.)
- Tamari (1 tsp.)

Preparation Technique:
1. Slice the brisket into strips. Mix the chili paste and stevia – stirring well.
2. Sprinkle the strips with tamari.
3. Heat a frying pan with the oil. Add the beef and prepare using the medium heat setting for ten minutes.
4. Blend in the stevia mixture and cook (medium heat setting) for another ten minutes.
5. Once the meat is tender, serve it.

Chicken Salad Deviled Eggs

Servings Provided: 6
Macro Counts - Per Serving:
- Net Carbs: 2 g
- Calories: 128
- Protein: 13 g
- Fat Content: 7 g

Ingredients:

- Chopped onion (1 tbsp.)

- Dijon mustard (1 tsp.)

- Mayonnaise (2 tbsp.)

- Old Bay Seasoning (1 dash)

- Lemon pepper (.5 tsp.)

- Dill (.5 tsp.)

- Celery salt (1 pinch)

- Shredded chicken (1 cup)

- Large eggs (6)

Preparation Technique:
1. Combine all of the fixings, omit the eggs, and store them in the fridge for later.
2. Gently place the eggs in a pot of water (enough to cover the eggs).
3. Set the temperature on high and wait for it to boil, and lower the setting to medium.
4. Boil for 15 minutes and chill them using cold running water.
5. Remove the shell and slice the eggs into halves.

6. Remove the yolk and fill it with the salad mixture. Sprinkle with the old bay seasoning and serve.
7. *Note*: The total time is just 30 minutes.

Coleslaw Stuffed Wraps

Servings Provided:4/16 wraps
Macro Counts - Per Serving:
- Net Carbs: 3 g
- Calories: 609
- Protein: 33 g
- Fat Content: 50 g

Ingredients:
- Sea salt (.25 tsp.)
- Green onions (.5 cup)
- Red cabbage (3 cups)
- Keto-friendly mayonnaise (.75 cup)
- Apple cider vinegar (2 tsp.)
    The Wraps & Other Fillings:
    - Ground beef/turkey/pork/chicken– cooked & chilled (1 lb.)
    - Collard leaves (16)
    - Packed alfalfa sprouts (.33 cup)
    - Toothpicks

Preparation Technique:
1. Prepare the meat of choice in a frying pan. Thinly slice the cabbage. Remove the stems from the collards and dice the onions. Add all of the fixings in a large mixing container and stir well.
2. Add a spoonful of the coleslaw on the far edge of the first collard leaf (the side that hasn't been cut). Add the meat and the sprouts.
3. Roll and tuck the sides and insert toothpicks at an angle to hold them together. Continue until all are done. Serve.

Grilled Caprese Skewers With Sourdough & Halloumi

Servings Provided:4-6

Macro Counts - Per Serving: The first set of grams is for the oil/the 2nd set is for the skewers with totals for both:

- Net Carbs: 0/25 g
- Calories: 108/308 = 416
- Protein: 0/15 g
- Fat Content: 12/17 = 29 g

Ingredients:

The Garlic Oil:

- Olive oil (.33 cup)
- Garlic (3 cloves)

The Skewers:

- Sourdough bread (3 cups)
- Halloumi (3 cups)
- Cherry tomatoes (4 cups)
- Salt and black pepper (as desired)
- Basil leaves (.75 cup)
- Balsamic vinegar (as needed)

Preparation Technique:
1. Thinly slice the garlic. Cube the halloumi and bread.
2. Prepare the oil and garlic using the med-low temperature setting for two to three minutes. Cool and remove the bits of garlic.
3. Prepare the skewers with two to three chunks of bread, three to four chunks of cheese, and three to four tomatoes per skewer.
4. Use the garlic oil and brush both sides of each skewer. Dust them with salt and pepper.
5. Prepare the grill and work the skewers in batches until nicely charred or two to three minutes on each side.
6. Add several leaves of basal to each end of the skewer and garnish with the chopped basil.
7. Serve with a drizzle of vinegar - immediately for the best results.

Lunch Kabobs

Servings Provided:6 kabobs
Macro Counts - Per Serving:
- Net Carbs: 4 g
- Calories: 214
- Protein: 8 g
- Fat Content: 17 g

Ingredients:
- Lunchmeat (12 slices)
- Lettuce (as desired)
- Black olives (12)
- Cherry tomatoes (12)
- Cheese (12 cubes)

Preparation Technique:
1. Prepare the fixings conveniently to make the skewers.
2. Layer each of the skewers the way you like them.
3. If you are not ready to serve quite yet, pop them in the fridge.

Roasted Cauliflower with Blue Cheese Sauce & Bacon

Servings Provided:4
Macro Counts - Per Serving:
- Net Carbs: 4 g
- Calories: 352
- Protein: 10 g
- Fat Content: 32 g

Ingredients:
- Cauliflower (1 head)
- Mayonnaise (.5 cup)
- Bacon crumbs (.5 cup)
- Blue cheese chunks (1 cup)

Preparation Technique:
1. Quarter the cauliflower and remove the stem and leaves.
2. Finely chop the blue cheese.
3. Preheat the oven to 350° Fahrenheit.
4. Spritz a baking tin with a misting of cooking oil spray. Arrange the cauliflower quarters on the baking pan. Roast for 30 minutes.
5. Meanwhile, make the sauce by combining the blue cheese and mayonnaise.
6. After 30 minutes, the cauliflower should be slightly tender.
7. Finish up by dressing the cauliflower with the blue cheese sauce.
8. Drizzle with the bacon bits.
9. Bake until the cheese sauce is golden or for 10 to 15 minutes.

Spinach Salmon Roulade

Servings Provided:18
Macro Counts - Per Serving:
- Net Carbs: 1 g
- Calories: 108
- Protein: 8 g
- Fat Content: 8 g

Ingredients:
- Smoked salmon (200 g - 7 slices)
- Eggs (3)
- Frozen spinach (200 g - 7 oz.)
- Hard cheese (200 g/2 cups)
- Cream cheese (200 g/1 cup)
- Caviar (100 g/6 tbsp.)

Preparation Technique:
1. Warm the oven to reach 400° Fahrenheit.
2. Use a hand blender to mix the eggs until fluffy and mix in the unfrozen spinach.
3. Add the mixture to a silicone sheet or baking tin lined with a sheet of parchment baking paper.
4. Spread it evenly and add the grated cheese over the top.
5. Bake the roulade for 15 minutes.
6. Cool it and add the cream cheese to the next layer. Arrange the slices of salmon over that.
7. Put a row of the caviar in a row where you begin rolling.
8. Roll them tightly to the end. Wrap it in cling wrap and twist the ends securely closed.
9. Pop it in the fridge (best results overnight). It's ready to serve when chilled.

Sushi

Servings Provided:3
Macro Counts - Per Serving:
- Net Carbs: 5.7 g
- Calories: 353
- Protein: 18 g
- Fat Content: 25.7 g

Ingredients:
- Smoked salmon/any seafood (5 oz.)
- Cauliflower (16 oz.)
- Cucumber (1 - 6-inches)
- Unchilled/softened cream cheese (6 oz.)
- Soy sauce/coconut aminos (1 tbsp.)
- Unseasoned rice vinegar (1-2 tbsp.)
- Nori sheets (5)
- Medium avocado (half of 1)
    - *Also Needed:*
- Food processor
- Bamboo roller

Preparation Technique:
1. Pulse the cauliflower into rice-sized bits. Set aside for now.
2. Cut up the cucumber first – end to end. Hold it upright and slice off each side. Trash the middle piece (or use it in for a fresh salad). Also, slice two side pieces into strips. Put it in the fridge.
3. Prepare a hot pan and cook the cauliflower rice. Sprinkle with approximately one tablespoon of the aminos.
4. When done, add the rice to a bowl with the cream cheese and vinegar. Stir well and place in the refrigerator.
5. Slice one-half of the avocado into strips. Scoop the shell.

6. Place a nori sheet on a bamboo roller covered with saran wrap. Spread the mixture on the nori sheet, add the fillings, and roll. Be sure it's tight.
7. Serve when it is ready.

Smoothies For A Quick Snack - Meal or Appetizer

Almond Lover Smoothie

Servings Provided:
Macro Counts - Per Serving:
- Net Carbs: 0 g
- Calories: 511
- Protein: 12 g
- Fat Content: 23 g

Ingredients:

- Almond milk (1 cup/8 oz.)

- Plain nonfat Greek yogurt (.33 cup)

- Cooked oats (.33 cup)

- Almonds (5)

- Medium banana (1)

- Almond butter (2 tbsp.)

Preparation Technique:
1. Measure all of the fixings into the cup of a NutriBullet or favorite high-speed machine.
2. Pour the milk up to the "max fill" line.
3. Blend until it is smooth and creamy.

Banana Bread & Blueberry Smoothie

Servings Provided:2
Macro Counts - Per Serving:
- Net Carbs: 4.7 g
- Calories: 270
- Protein: 3.1 g
- Fat Content: 23.3 g

Ingredients:

- Chia seeds (1 tbsp.)

- Golden flaxseed meal (3 tbsp.)

- Vanilla unsweetened coconut milk (2 cups)

- Blueberries (.25 cup)

- Liquid stevia (10 drops)

- MCT oil (2 tbsp.

- Xanthan gum (.25 tsp.)

- Banana extract (1.5 tsp.)

- Ice cubes (2-3)

Preparation Technique:
1. Combine all of the ingredients into a blender.
2. Wait a few minutes for the seeds and flax to absorb some of the liquid.
3. Pulse for 1-2 minutes until well combined and the texture you choose. Lastly, add the ice to your preference.

Keto Avocado-Raspberry Smoothie

Servings Provided: 2
Macro Counts - Per Serving:
- Net Carbs: 4 g
- Calories: 227
- Protein: 2.5 g
- Fat Content: 20 g

Ingredients:

- Ripe avocado (1)

- Lemon juice (3 tbsp.)

- Water (1.33 cups)

- Frozen unsweetened raspberries/or choice of berries (.5 cup)

- Your preference of a sugar equivalent (1 tbsp. + 1 tsp.)

Preparation Technique:
1. Chop the avocado into chunks.
2. Toss each of the fixings into a blender and mix until it's smooth.
3. Pour the smoothie into two glasses and serve.
4. Note: You can choose other berries, but be sure to calculate any additional carbs.

Strawberry Almond Smoothies

Servings Provided:2
Macro Counts - Per Serving:
- Net Carbs: 7 g
- Calories: 304
- Protein: 15 g
- Fat Content: 25 g

Ingredients:

- Frozen unsweetened strawberries (.25 cup)

- Unsweetened almond milk (16 oz.)

- Heavy cream (.5 cup)

- Stevia (to your liking)

- Whey vanilla isolate powder (2 tbsp.)

Preparation Technique:
1. Measure and add all of the fixings into a blender.
2. Pulse the components until it's as you like it to serve!

Chapter 6: Seafood & Poultry Specialties

Seafood Favorites

Blue Crabs with Lime - Chipotle & Brown Butter Sauce

Servings Provided:3
Macro Counts - Per Serving:
- Net Carbs: 10 g
- Calories: 349
- Protein: 16 g
- Fat Content: 31 g

Ingredients:
- Blue crabs (1 dozen - live)
- Crab boil seasoning (1 pkg.)
- Butter (.5 cup)
- Chopped red chilis (1 tsp.)
- Chopped chipotles (1 tbsp. canned)
- Ground coriander (1 tbsp.)
- Cayenne pepper (1 tsp.)
- Black pepper & salt (as desired)
- Fresh lime juice (2 tbsp.)
- Chopped cilantro (.25 cup)

Preparation Technique:

1. Prepare a crab pot with eight to ten quarts of water. Wait for it to boil. Add the seasonings. Grab the tongs to add the crabs - one at a time.
2. Dip them in (face first). Simmer for about ten minutes.
3. Meanwhile, prep a sauté pan with butter. Whisk in the cayenne, coriander, and chipotles. Sauté them for about four minutes or until they're lightly browned.
4. Set the pan off of the burner and add the lime juice, chopped chilis, and cilantro with a shake of pepper and salt.
5. Remove the crabs and add them to the sauce, stirring to cover each one.
6. Serve with a wedge of lemon.

Broiled Oyster with Spicy Sauce

Servings Provided:2
Macro Counts - Per Serving:
- Net Carbs: 2 g
- Calories: 102
- Protein: 4 g
- Fat Content: 8 g

Ingredients:
- Oysters (1 dozen)
- Garlic chili paste - ex. Huy Fong's (1 tbsp.)
- Olive oil (1 tbsp.)
- Salt (.125 tsp.)
- Fresh basil (7-8 leaves)

Preparation Technique:
1. Warm the oven using the broil function.
2. Shuck the oysters.
3. Prepare the garlic chili paste, salt, and oil. Add the oysters and toss to coat them.
4. Sprinkle the leaves of basil onto an oven-safe baking dish and add the oysters
5. Empty the sauce into the dish.
6. Transfer the dish to the oven (top rack) and broil on high for two to three minutes and serve right away.

Cajun Trinity Keto Crab Cakes

Servings Provided:8 cakes/2 per serving
Macro Counts - Per Serving:
- Net Carbs: 3 g
- Calories: 412
- Protein: 35 g
- Fat Content: 28 g

Ingredients:
- Butter (2 tbsp.)
- Celery (1 large rib)
- Mixed bell pepper (.5 cup)
- Shallot (1)
- Garlic (2 cloves)
- Sea salt and black pepper (as desired)
- Large egg (1)
- Keto-friendly mayo (2 tbsp.)
- Worcestershire sauce (1 tbsp.)
- Spicy brown mustard (1 tsp.)
- Hot sauce (1 tsp.)
- Parmesan cheese (.5 cup)
- Crushed pork rinds (.5 cup)
- Lump crabmeat (1 lb.)
- Olive oil (2 tbsp.)

Preparation Technique:

1. Warm a large skillet/sauté pan using the medium temperature setting.
2. Chop/dice the celery, shallot, garlic, and peppers. Toss them into the pan and sauté them for about ten minutes.
3. Combine the mayo, egg, Worcestershire sauce, hot sauce, and mustard. Mix in the sautéed veggies and stir well.
4. Fold in the parmesan and pork rinds along with the crab mixture.
5. Prepare a baking tray/large platter with a sheet of parchment paper and make eight patties.
6. Pop them in the fridge for one to two hours.
7. Warm a skillet (med-high temperature) and add the oil.
8. Fry the patties until browned - not flipping too frequently, or they may break apart.

Chaffles & Prawns with Toppings

Servings Provided:3
Macro Counts - Per Serving:
- Net Carbs: 1.14 g
- Calories: 158
- Protein: 17.3 g
- Fat Content: 8.4 g

Ingredients:
- Large egg (1)
- Almond flour (1 tbsp.)
- Full-fat Greek yogurt (1 tbsp.)
- Shredded Swiss cheese (.25 cup)
- Baking powder (.125 tsp.)
    - *The Topping*:
- Grilled prawns (4 oz.)
- Steamed cauliflower mash (4 oz.)
- Sliced zucchini (half of 1)
- Tomato (1 sliced)
- Flaxseeds (1 tbsp.)
- Lettuce leaves (3 large leaves)

Preparation Technique:
1. Toss the chaffles fixings in a bowl and mix thoroughly.
2. Heat the waffle maker. Prepare the chaffles in three batches, cooking for three to four minutes until they are crispy.
3. When ready, arrange the leaves of lettuce, and the rest of the toppings to serve.

Cioppino Italian Seafood Stew - Gluten-Free

Servings Provided:6
Macro Counts - Per Serving:
- Net Carbs: 7 g
- Calories: 284
- Protein: 23 g
- Fat Content: 11 g

Ingredients:
- Olive oil (2 tbsp.)
- Butter (2 tbsp.)
- Onion (1)
- Carrot (1)
- Celery (2 stalks)
- Sea salt
- Garlic (5 cloves)
- White wine (2 cups)
- Gluten-free crushed tomatoes (28 oz. can)
- Fish stock/clam juice (1.5 cups)
- Dried oregano (1 tsp.)
- Old Bay Seasoning (1 tsp.)
- Red pepper flakes (.5 tsp.
- Worcestershire sauce (1 tsp.)
- Anchovy paste (1 tbsp.)
- Lemon juice (2 tsp.)
- Cod/halibut (8 oz.)
- Shrimp (16-20 or ¾ lb.)
- Raw mussels (1 lb.)
- Raw clams (1 dozen)
- Freshly chopped basil (2 tbsp.)

Preparation Technique:
1. Cut the chosen fish into two-inch chunks. Peel and devein the shrimp.
2. Warm a dutch oven using the med-low temperature setting. Melt the olive oil with the butter.

3. Mince or dice the celery, onions, garlic, and carrot. Toss them in the pot with salt. Sauté them for about five minutes. (Toss in the garlic for the last minute.)
4. Raise the setting to high and pour in the wine. Simmer for two minutes and add the fish stock, crushed tomatoes, Worcestershire sauce, anchovy paste, oregano, red pepper flakes, and Old Bay.
5. Lower the setting to low and continue to simmer for 20 more minutes.
6. Bring it to a boil and add the pieces of cod, lemon juice, and shrimp. Cook for three minutes. Remove the shrimp and set them aside for now.
7. Add the clams and mussels (in the shell). Place a lid on the pot and simmer until the shellfish have opened. (6 min.).
8. Toss the shrimp back in the pot with pepper and salt.
9. Serve with a portion of chopped basil.

Crunchy Fish and Chaffle Bites

Servings Provided:4
Macro Counts - Per Serving:
- Net Carbs: 1.3 g
- Calories: 321
- Protein: 28.7g
- Fat Content: 21.4 g

Ingredients:
- Cod fillets (1 lb./4 slices)
- Garlic powder (1 tsp.)
- Sea salt (1 tsp.)
- Whisked egg (1)
- Almond flour (1 cup)
- Avocado oil (2 tsp.)
  The Chaffles:
- Cheddar cheese (.5 cup)
- Eggs (2)
- Italian seasoning (.5 tsp.)
- Almond flour (2 tbsp.)

Preparation Technique:
1. Whisk the chaffle fixings and warm the mini waffle maker.
2. Pour the batter into the heated waffle iron.
3. Whisk the garlic powder, pepper, and salt. Add the cod to the mixture and wait for about ten minutes.
4. At that point, dip them into the almond flour.
5. Warm the oil in a skillet and fry the fish for two to three minutes. Serve the delicious fish with the chaffles.

Lemon Butter Scallops

Servings Provided:4
Macro Counts - Per Serving:
- Net Carbs: 5 g
- Calories: 289
- Protein: 15.9 g
- Fat Content: 22.7 g

Ingredients:
- Butter (4 tbsp. - divided)
- Scallops (1 lb.)
- Lemon zest & juice (1 lemon)
- Pepper and salt (to your liking)

Preparation Technique:
1. Rinse the scallops under cold tap water and pat dry. Season with the pepper and salt.
2. Slice the lemon in half, using for the juice and half for the zest.
3. Over the medium-high heat setting, melt two tablespoons of the butter. Toss in the scallops and prepare for five to seven minutes per side.
4. Once they're crispy, squeeze half of the freshly squeezed lemon juice over the scallops and add to a serving dish.
5. Add the rest of the butter to the skillet and blend in the rest of the lemon juice and lemon zest. Stir it for four to five minutes or until the butter is slightly reduced.
6. The leftovers are good for up to two days if stored in an airtight container.

Mahi-Mahi Fillets

Servings Provided: 4
Macro Counts - Per Serving:
- Net Carbs: 0 g
- Calories: 200
- Protein: 21 g
- Fat Content: 13 g

Ingredients:
- Butter - divided (3 tbsp.)
- Olive oil - divided (2 tbsp.)
- Mahi-mahi fillets (4 - 4 oz.)
- Black pepper and kosher salt (as desired)
- Asparagus (1 lb.)
- Garlic (3 cloves)
- Red pepper flakes (.25 tsp.)
- Lemon (1 sliced/zest and juice)
- Freshly chopped parsley (1 tbsp. + more for garnish)

Preparation Technique:
1. Prepare a large skillet using the medium temperature setting and add one tablespoon each of oil and butter. Arrange the fish in the pan with a dusting of salt and pepper. Cook it until it is golden or about four to five minutes on each side. Plate it for now.
2. Pour the rest of the oil into the skillet. Toss in the asparagus with salt and pepper, and sauté until it's tender (2 to 4 min.). Transfer it to a plate.
3. Add the remaining two tablespoons of butter to the skillet. Mince and add the garlic, pepper flakes, lemon juice, zest, and parsley.
4. Take the pan off of the burner and add back the fish, asparagus, and sauce to the skillet.
5. Serve with parsley as desired.

Pan-Fried Cod

Servings Provided:4
Macro Counts - Per Serving:
- Net Carbs: 1 g
- Calories: 160
- Fat Content: 7 g
- Protein: 21 g

Ingredients:
- Garlic cloves (6)
- Ghee (3 tbsp.)
- Cod fillets (4 @ ⅓ lb. ea.)
- *Optional:* Garlic powder

Preparation Technique:
1. Mince the garlic and toss half of it into a skillet with the ghee.
2. Arrange the fillets in the pan using medium-high heat. Sprinkle them using the garlic, and if desired, a portion of pepper and salt.
3. Once it turns white halfway up its side, turn it over, and add the remainder of the minced garlic. Continue cooking until it flakes easily.
4. Serve with a portion of ghee or garlic from the pan.

Shrimp Alfredo

Servings Provided:4
Macro Counts - Per Serving:

- Net Carbs: 6.5 g
- Calories: 298
- Protein: 23 g
- Fat Content: 18 g

Ingredients:

- Raw shrimp (1 lb.)
- Salted butter (1 tbsp.)
- Cubed cream cheese (4 oz.)
- Whole milk (.5 cup)
- Salt (1 tsp.)
- Dried basil (1 tsp.)
- Garlic powder (1 tbsp.)
- Shredded parmesan cheese (.5 cup)
- Baby kale or spinach (.25 cup)
- Whole sun-dried tomatoes (5)

Preparation Technique:

1. Heat the butter using the medium heat setting in a skillet.
2. Toss in the shrimp and lower the heat to medium-low. After 30 seconds, flip the shrimp and cook until slightly pink. Blend in the cream cheese.
3. Increase the heat and pour in the milk. Stir frequently.
4. Sprinkle with the salt, basil, and garlic. Empty the parmesan cheese in and mix well.
5. Simmer until the sauce has thickened. Cut the sun-dried tomatoes into strips.
6. Lastly, fold in the kale/spinach and dried tomatoes. Serve steaming hot.

Shrimp & Bacon Risotto

Servings Provided:2
Macro Counts - Per Serving:
- Net Carbs: 5 g
- Calories: 224
- Protein: 24 g
- Fat Content: 9 g

Ingredients:
- Bacon (4 slices)
- Daikon winter radish (2 cups)
- Dry white wine (2 tbsp.)
- Chicken stock (.25 cup)
- Garlic (1 clove)
- Ground pepper (as desired)
- Chopped parsley (2 tbsp.)
- Cooked shrimp (4 oz.)

Preparation Technique:
1. Peel and slice the radish, mince the garlic, and chop the bacon. Remove as much water as possible from the daikon once it's shredded.
2. On the stovetop, warm a saucepan using the medium heat temperature setting. Toss in the bacon and fry until it's crispy. Leave the drippings in the pan and remove the bacon with a slotted spoon to drain.
3. Add the stock, wine, daikon, salt, pepper, and garlic into the pan. Simmer until most of the liquid is absorbed (6-8 min.).
4. Fold in the bacon (saving a few bits for the topping), and shrimp along with the parsley. Serve.
5. *Tip*: If you cannot find the daikon, substitute it using shredded cauliflower.

Tuna Fritter

Servings Provided: 3
Macro Counts - Per Serving:
- Net Carbohydrates: 2.9 g
- Calories: 106
- Protein: 1.1 g
- Fat Content: 10.5 g

Ingredients:
- Chunks of tuna (.5 cup)
- Almond flour (3 tbsp.)
- Mayonnaise (2 tbsp.)
- Grated cheese (2 tbsp.)
- Onion (2 tbsp.)
- Garlic powder (.5 tsp. each)
- Salt and pepper (.25 tsp. each)
- Red pepper flakes (1 tsp.)
- Coconut oil (2 tbsp.)

Preparation Technique:
1. Break the tuna into chunks using a fork and mix with the mayonnaise, grated cheese, and chopped onion.
2. Make the mixture into patties and sprinkle with the pepper flakes, garlic powder, pepper, and salt.
3. Coat the patties with the flour and add to a hot skillet with the coconut oil using the low heat setting.
4. Cook about three minutes, turn the patties over and continue cooking until browned (approximately another three minutes). Serve.

Poultry Options

Asparagus-Stuffed Chicken

Servings Provided:4
Macro Counts - Per Serving:
- Net Carbs: 2 g
- Calories: 377
- Protein: 32 g
- Fat Content: 25 g

Ingredients:
- Bacon pieces (.5 lb. or 8 slices)
- Chicken tenders (8 or about 1 lb.)
- Black pepper (.25 tsp)
- Salt (.5 tsp.)
- Asparagus spears (12/about .5 lb.)

Preparation Technique:
1. Set the oven to reach 400° Fahrenheit.
2. Prepare a baking sheet and lay out two slices of bacon.
3. Arrange the chicken tenders on top of that and sprinkle with a dusting of pepper and salt.
4. Add three spears of the asparagus and wrap with the bacon and chicken to hold it all together.
5. Continue the process and bake for 40 minutes. The bacon should be crispy and the asparagus tender.

Bacon-Wrapped Chicken - Air Fryer

Servings Provided:3
Macro Counts - Per Serving:
- Net Carbohydrates: 0.6 g
- Calories: 364
- Protein: 31 g
- Fat Content: 26 g

Ingredients:
- Breast of chicken (1)
- Unsmoked bacon (6 strips)
- Soft garlic cheese (1 tbsp.)

Preparation Technique:
1. Slice the chicken into six pieces. Spread the garlic cheese over each strip of bacon. Add a bit of chicken to each one.
2. Roll and secure with a toothpick.
3. Warm the Air Fryer for 3-4 minutes. Arrange the wraps in the heated Air Fryer and cook 15 minutes for a quick snack at any time.

Chicken Enchilada Bowl

Servings Provided:4
Macro Counts - Per Serving:
- Net Carbs: 6 g
- Calories: 569
- Protein: 39 g
- Fat Content: 40 g

Ingredients:
- Coconut oil (2 tbsp.)
- Skinless - boneless chicken thighs (1 lb.)
- Water (.25 cup)
- Red enchilada sauce (.75 cup)
- Chopped onion (.25 cup)
- Diced green chiles (4 oz. can)
  The Toppings:
- Avocado (1 whole - diced)
- Sour cream (.5 cup)
- Shredded cheese (1 cup)
- Chopped pickled jalapenos (.25 cup)
- Roma tomato (1 chopped)
- *Optional*: Serve over plain cauliflower rice or Mexican cauliflower rice

Preparation Technique:
1. Melt the coconut oil in a large pot using the medium heat setting.
2. Sear the chicken until lightly browned.
3. Empty the water and enchilada sauce. Toss in the green chiles and onion.
4. Reduce the temperature and simmer. Prepare the chicken for 17 to 25 temperature minutes.
5. When the chicken reaches 165° Fahrenheit - internally remove and cool slightly.
6. Shred or chop the meat and toss it back into the pot.
7. Simmer for another ten minutes so the sauce will reduce in volume.

8. To serve, top with the jalapeno, avocado, tomato, cheese, sour cream, and any other desired toppings.
9. Note: Serve over a portion of cauliflower rice or any other desired topping making sure to add any additional carbs used.

Chicken Mozzarella & Pesto Casserole

Servings Provided: 8
Macro Counts - Per Serving:
- Net Carbs: 3 g
- Calories: 451
- Protein: 38 g
- Fat Content: 30 g

Ingredients:
- Cooking oil (as needed)
- Grilled & cubed chicken breasts (2 lb.)
- Unchilled cream cheese (8 oz.)
- Cubed & Shredded mozzarella (8 oz. of each)
- Pesto (.25 cup)
- Heavy cream (.25 to .5 cup)

Preparation Technique:
1. Heat the oven to reach 400° Fahrenheit. Spritz a casserole dish using a cooking oil spray.
2. Combine the heavy cream, pesto, and softened cream cheese.
3. Add the chicken and cubed mozzarella into the greased dish.
4. Bake it for 25 to 30 minutes.
5. *Cooking Tip*: Use ½ cup of cream if you prefer a thinner sauce or ¼ cup for a thicker choice.

Chicken Parmesan Meatballs

Servings Provided:4
Macro Counts - Per Serving:
- Net Carbs: 3 g
- Calories: 257
- Protein: 26 g
- Fat Content: 15 g

Ingredients:
- Three Cheese Garlic Marinara Sauce (.5 cup)
- Ground chicken (1 lb.)
- Minced garlic (3 cloves)
- Grated parmesan cheese (.25 cup)
- Chopped fresh flat-leaf parsley (3 tbsp.)
- Dried Italian seasoning (.5 tsp.)
- Onion powder (.5 tsp.)
- Sea salt (.5 tsp.)
- Black pepper (.25 tsp.)
- Shredded mozzarella cheese (.5 cup)

Preparation Technique:
1. Heat the oven to reach 350° Fahrenheit
2. Lightly grease a large baking dish.
3. In a large mixing container, combine two tablespoons of the marinara sauce, the ground chicken, parsley, onion powder, garlic, parmesan cheese, Italian seasoning, salt, and pepper
4. Shape the mixture into twelve meatballs.
5. Arrange the prepared meatballs in the baking dish. Leave a small space between each meatball.
6. Bake on the center rack of the oven for 25 minutes.
7. Place the dish on the countertop. Pour in the rest of the sauce over the top of the balls in the pan.
8. Cover the meatballs with mozzarella cheese.
9. Set the oven temperature setting to broil.

10. Once it is hot, place the meatballs back in the oven
    until the cheese is melted and golden brown or
    approximately two to three minutes.

Chicken Tenders - Chick-fil-A Copycat

Servings: 8 tenders
Total Time Required: 25 Minutes
Macro Counts - Per Serving:
- Net Carbohydrates: 0.5 g
- Calories: 104
- Protein: 26.8 g
- Fat Content: 9 g

Ingredients:
- Chicken tenders (8)
- Dill pickle juice (24 oz. jar)
- Almond flour (.75 cup)
- Salt and pepper (1 tsp. of each)
- Eggs (2 beaten)
- Breadcrumb substitute ex. Pork panko (1.5 cups)
- For Frying: Nutiva Organic Coconut Oil
  The Sauce:
- Yellow mustard (2 tsp.)
- Mayo (.5 cup)
- Lemon Juice (1 tsp.)
- Honey Trees Sugar-Free Honey (2 tbsp.)
- BBQ sauce - ex. Organicville (1 tbsp.)

Preparation Technique:
1. Put the chicken tenders and pickle juice in a sizable zipper-type bag and marinate for at least one hour (overnight is recommended).
2. Sift the almond flour, pepper, and salt.
3. Prepare three bowls: #1 Almond flour mixture; #2 - eggs, and #3 - pork panko
4. Dredge the chicken in the almond flour mixture, egg, and pork panko until thoroughly coated.
5. Prepare a skillet with about two inches of coconut oil (med-high temperature).
6. Once the oil is hot, place the tenders in the pan and cook them until golden brown (3 min. per side).

For An Air Fryer:
1. Set the Air Fryer at 375° Fahrenheit.
2. Cook the chicken for about 15 minutes.

Creamy Onion Chicken

Servings Provided:4
Macro Counts - Per Serving:

- Net Carbs: 3 g
- Calories: 400
- Protein: 38 g
- Fat Content: 26 g

Ingredients:

- Whole green spring onion (1)
- Butter (2 tbsp. or 1 oz.)
- Chicken breast halves (4)
- Sour cream (8 oz.)
- Sea salt (.5 tsp.)

Preparation Technique:

1. Remove all skin and bones from the chicken breasts.
2. Warm a skillet using the med-high setting to melt the butter.
3. Reduce the setting to med-low and arrange the chicken in the skillet with the butter. Place a lid on the pan and cook for about ten minutes.
4. Chop the onion using the white and green sections. Flip the chicken breasts. Cover and simmer for another eight or nine minutes or until done.
5. Combine the onion and cook an additional one or two minutes.
6. Take it off the burner. Blend in the sour cream and salt.
7. Wait for about five minutes. Mix well with your favorite veggies and serve.

Kung Pao Chicken

Servings Provided:4
Macro Counts - Per Serving:
- Net Carbohydrates: 4 g
- Calories: 264
- Protein: 23 g
- Fat Content: 18 g

Ingredients:
The Chicken:
- Coconut oil (1 tbsp.)
- Red bell pepper (.33 of 1 medium)
- Celery (2 stalks)
- Peanuts (.25 cup)
- Ground ginger (1 tsp.)
- Minced garlic (.5 tsp.)
- Chicken thighs (4 skinless/boneless)
- *Optional:* Xanthan Gum (.25 tsp.)
  The Sauce:
- Liquid aminos (.25 cup)
- Chicken broth (.25 cup)
- Chili garlic sauce/sriracha sauce (1.5 tbsp.)
- Sesame oil (1 tsp.)
- Liquid stevia (30 drops)
- Rice wine vinegar (1 tsp.)

Preparation Technique:
1. Dice the celery stalks and bell pepper into big chunks and set aside.
2. Heat a large skillet using the med-high temperature setting.
3. Chop the thighs into bite-sized chunks.
4. Pour in the coconut oil to the hot skillet and toss in the chunks of chicken.
5. Prepare the sauce while the chicken is cooking. Combine all of the sauce fixings in a mixing container. Whisk well and set to the side for now.

6. Once the chicken is almost fully cooked, fold in the veggies.
7. Simmer until they are slightly tender (2-3 min.).
8. Fold in the peanuts and continue to cook for another few minutes while they toast.
9. Add in the ginger and garlic. Stir once more and add in the sauce.
10. Continue cooking and add the xanthan gum to thicken up the sauce even more.
11. Serve with cauliflower rice or on its own.

Lemon Parsley Buttered Chicken - Slow Cooked

Servings Provided:6
Macro Counts - Per Serving:
- Net Carbs: 1 g
- Calories: 300
- Protein: 29 g
- Fat Content: 18 g

Ingredients:
- Whole roasting chicken (5-6 lb.)
- Black pepper (.25 tsp.)
- Kosher salt (.5 tsp.)
- Water (1 cup)
- Thinly sliced lemon (1)
- Ghee/butter (4 tbsp.)
- Chopped fresh parsley (2 tbsp.)

Preparation Technique:
1. Remove the innards (discard) and rinse the chicken. Dry it off with some paper towels and rub it with the pepper and salt.
2. Arrange the whole chicken in the slow cooker and pour the water into the pot. Set the cooker for 3 hours or when the bird reaches an internal temperature of 165° Fahrenheit at the thickest segment of the thigh.
3. Add the lemon slices, butter, and parsley into the cooker for about ten minutes.
4. *To Serve*: Pour the parsley butter over the chicken and enjoy. Garnish with other toppings of your choosing.

Chapter 7: Pork & Beef

Pork

Kalua Pork & Cabbage

Servings Provided:12
Macro Counts - Per Serving:
- Net Carbs: 4 g
- Calories: 227
- Protein: 22 g
- Fat Content: 13 g

Ingredients:
- Head of cabbage (1 medium - 2 lb.)
- Bacon (7 strips - divided)
- Boneless pork shoulder butt (3 lb.)
- Coarse sea salt (1 tbsp.)
- *Suggested*: 6-quart slow cooker

Preparation Technique:
1. Coarsely chop the cabbage. Trim the fat from the roast.
2. Layer most of the bacon in the cooker. Dust the salt over the roast and place the rest of the bacon on top. Close the lid and cook on low for eight to ten hours.
3. At that time, add in the cabbage and continue cooking with the pot covered for another hour or until it's tender. (Times may vary.)
4. When the roast is done, remove and shred it. Use a slotted spoon to arrange the cabbage in the serving dish.
5. Use a portion of the slow cooker juices on the side for dipping.

Pork-Chop Onion & Mushroom Fat Bombs

Servings Provided: 3
Macro Counts - Per Serving:
- Net Carbs: 7 g
- Calories: 1076
- Protein: 30 g
- Fat Content: 103 g

Ingredients:
- Boneless pork chops (3)
- Oil (.5 cup)
- Medium yellow onion (1)
- Brown mushrooms (8 oz.)
- Nutmeg (1 tsp.)
- Garlic powder (1 tsp.)
- Balsamic vinegar (1 tbsp.)
- Mayonnaise (1 cup)

Preparation Technique:
1. Rinse, drain, and slice the mushrooms. Peel and slice the onion. Put them in a large skillet with the oil and sauté until wilted.
2. Place the chops to the side and sprinkle with the nutmeg and garlic powder. Cook until done. Transfer the prepared chops onto a plate.
3. Whisk in the vinegar and mayonnaise into the pan. The thick sauce can be thinned with a bit of chicken broth if needed. (Add two tablespoons at a time.)
4. Ladle the sauce over the bomb and serve.

Pork Kebabs

Servings Provided:4
Macro Counts - Per Serving:
- Net Carbs: 3.3 g
- Protein: 34 g
- Fat Content: 9 g

Ingredients:

- Hot sauce (2 tsp.)

- Sunflower seed butter (3 tbsp.)

- Minced garlic (1 tbsp.)

- Keto-friendly soy sauce (1 tbsp.)

- Water (1 tbsp.)

- Medium green pepper (1)

- Crushed red pepper (.5 tsp.)

- Squared pork for kebabs (1 lb.)

Preparation Technique:
1. Heat the oven or grill using the broil or the high heat setting.
2. In a processor/blender, combine the water with the red pepper, butter, soy sauce, garlic, and hot sauce.
3. Slice the pork into squares. Cover with the marinade and rest for one hour.
4. Chop the peppers to fit the skewer. Thread the skewers alternating the pork and peppers.
5. Broil using the high heat setting for five minutes per side.

Stuffed Pork Chops

Servings Provided:4
Macro Counts - Per Serving:
- Net Carbs: 1 g
- Calories: 778
- Protein: 102 g
- Fat Content: 38 g

Ingredients:
- Bacon (3 slices)
- Thick-cut pork chops (4)
- Blue cheese (3 oz.)
- Cream cheese (2 oz.)
- Feta cheese (3 oz.)
- Green onion (.33 cup)
- Garlic powder (1 pinch)
- Black pepper and salt (to taste)

Preparation Technique:
1. Set the oven temperature to 350° Fahrenheit. Lightly grease a baking tin.
2. Prepare the bacon, reserving the grease, and set aside.
3. Mix the feta and blue cheese. Blend in the onions, bacon, and cream cheese. Mix well.
4. Split the non-fat side of the pork and add the cheese mixture – closing with a toothpick or skewer. Sprinkle using the salt, pepper, and garlic powder.
5. Sear them using the bacon grease in the skillet for 1.5 minutes per side.
6. Arrange the chops on the baking pan and cook for 55 minutes. Wait for the chops to rest for about three minutes.

Beef

Keto chaffle recipes are the new trend to dieting using the ketogenic diet plan. They are extremely simple to prepare and can be used as bread for a sandwich, burger, pizza, and dessert. The ketogenic diet program is excellent for helping you lose weight and be provided with many benefits in the meanwhile. Let's break it down, so you better understand what chaffles are and how they fit into your dieting techniques with one beef and one fish chaffle (check the seafood section)!

Sloppy Joe Chaffles

Servings Provided:4
Macro Counts - Per Serving:
- Net Carbs: 2.7 g
- Calories: 156
- Protein: 26 g
- Fat Content:3.9 g

Ingredients:
- Ground beef (1 lb.)
- Onion powder (1 tsp.) or Regular onion (.25 cup)
- Garlic (1 tsp.)
- Tomato paste (3 tbsp.)
- Salt (.5 tsp.)
- Pepper (.25 tsp.)
- Chili powder (1 tbsp.)
- Optional: Cocoa powder (1 tsp.)
- Bone broth - beef flavor usually (.5 cup)
- Coconut aminos (1 tsp.)
- Mustard powder (1 tsp.)
- Swerve brown/Sukrin golden (1 tsp.)
- Paprika (.5 tsp.)

Preparation Technique:
1. Cook the ground beef with salt and pepper first.

2. Mince the garlic and add all the rest of the fixings and simmer.
3. Preheat waffle iron.
4. Whip the egg and add the remaining ingredients.
5. Spray the waffle maker with nonstick cooking spray.
6. Divide the mixture in half and cook half the mixture for about four minutes or until golden brown.
7. For a crispy outer crust on the chaffle, add one teaspoon of cheese to the waffle maker for 30 seconds before adding the mixture.
8. Pour the warm sloppy joe mix onto a hot chaffle, and dinner is served!

Air Fryer Korean Tacos

Servings Provided:6
Macro Counts - Per Serving:
- Net Carbs: 8 g
- Calories: 241
- Protein: 27 g
- Fat Content: 10 g

Ingredients:
The Marinade:
- Gochujang (2 tbsp.)
- Dark soy sauce (1 tbsp.)
- Fresh garlic & ginger (2 tsp. of each)
- Sugar substitute/Truvia (1 tsp. - equivalent to 2 tsp. sugar)
- Sesame oil (2 tbsp.)
- Sesame seeds (2 tbsp.)
- Kosher salt (.5 tsp.)
    Meat & Veggies:
- Sirloin beef/chuck/or ribeye (1.5 lb.)
- Sliced onion (1 cup)
    To Serve:
- Flour tortillas (1 dozen)
- Romaine lettuce leaves (1 head)
- Chopped green scallions (.5 cup - into 2-inch pieces)
    Optional:
- Kimchi (.5 cup
- Cilantro (.25 cup)

Preparation Technique:

1. Thinly slice the beef. Mince the ginger and garlic. Chop the scallions and slice the onions.
2. Toss the onions, beef, in a zipper-type bag with soy sauce, gochujang, garlic, ginger, sesame oil, sweetener, and sesame seeds. "Squish" the bag to fully mix the ingredients.
3. Marinate it in the fridge for half an hour or as long as 24 hours.
4. Warm the Air Fryer to reach 400° Fahrenheit. When it's ready, add the veggies and meat in the fryer basket and cook for 12 minutes. Shake the basket about halfway through the cooking cycle.
5. Serve it when desired.
6. Note: You can also use this recipe with a pork shoulder for a bit of change!

Cabbage & Bacon Burger Stir Fry

Servings Provided: 10
Macro Counts - Per Serving:
- Net Carbs: 4.5 g
- Calories: 357
- Protein: 32 g
- Fat Content: 22 g

Ingredients:
- Ground beef (1 lb.)
- Bacon (1 lb.)
- Small onion (1)
- Minced cloves of garlic (3)
- Cabbage (1 lb. - 1 small head)
- Black pepper (.25 tsp.)
- Sea salt (.5 tsp.)

Preparation Technique:
1. Dice the bacon and onion.
2. Combine the beef and bacon in a wok or large skillet. Prepare until done and store in a bowl to keep warm.
3. Mince the onion and garlic. Toss both into the hot grease.
4. Slice and toss in the cabbage and stir-fry until wilted.
5. Blend in the meat and combine. Sprinkle with the pepper and salt as desired.

Cheeseburger Calzone

Servings Provided: 8
Macro Counts - Per Serving:
- Net Carbs: 3 g
- Calories: 580
- Protein: 34 g
- Fat Content: 47 g

Ingredients:
- Dill pickle spears (4)
- Yellow diced onion (half of 1)
- Ground beef – lean (1.5 lb.)
- Thick-cut bacon strips (4)
- Almond flour (1 cup)
- Cream cheese – divided (8 oz.)
- Shredded cheddar cheese (1 cup)
- Egg (1)
- Mayonnaise (.5 cup)
- Shredded mozzarella cheese (1 cup)

Preparation Technique:
1. Heat the oven to reach 425° Fahrenheit. Prepare a cookie tin with parchment paper.
2. Chop the pickles into spears. Set aside for now.
3. Prepare the crust. Combine half of the cream cheese and the mozzarella cheese. Microwave them for 35 seconds. When it melts, add the egg and almond flour to make the dough. Set aside.
4. Cook the beef on the stove using medium heat.
5. Cook the bacon (microwave for five minutes or on the stovetop). When cool, break into bits.
6. Dice the onion and add to the beef and cook until softened. Toss in the bacon, cheddar cheese, pickle bits, the rest of the cream cheese, and mayonnaise. Stir well.
7. Roll the dough onto the prepared baking tin. Scoop the mixture into the center. Fold the ends and side to

make the calzone.

8. Bake until browned or about 15 minutes. Let it rest for
   ten minutes before slicing.

Cheeseburger Spaghetti Squash Casserole

Servings Provided: 6
Macro Counts - Per Serving:
- Net Carbs: 6.5 g
- Calories: 431
- Protein: 30.5 g
- Fat Content: 28.8 g

Ingredients:
- Medium spaghetti squash (1)
- Bacon (4 slices)
- Ground beef (1 lb.)
- Cloves of garlic (2)
- Salt and pepper (.5 tsp.)
- Sugar-free ketchup (2 tbsp.)
- Worcestershire sauce (2 tsp.)
- Shredded cheddar (6 oz./about 1.5 cups)

Preparation Technique:

1. Warm the oven in advance to reach 400° Fahrenheit. Line a baking tray using a layer of parchment baking paper.
2. Cut the squash in half crosswise and scoop out the seeds. Arrange it cut-side down and bake until the squash is soft enough to be squeezed (40 min.).
3. Meanwhile, fry the bacon in a large skillet using the medium temperature setting until it's crispy. Transfer it to a paper towel-lined plate.
4. In the same skillet, cook the ground beef.
5. In about seven minutes, mince and the garlic, salt, and pepper. Cook until no longer pink (2-3 min.).
6. Stir in the ketchup and Worcestershire sauce. Scoop the flesh out of the squash and stir in until well mixed into the ground beef. Spread out evenly over the bottom of the skillet.
7. Sprinkle with the shredded cheddar cheese and cover the skillet.
8. Reduce the heat to low and let the cheese melt(5 min.).
9. Sprinkle the bacon over the top and serve.

Garlic Butter Prime Rib Roast

Servings Provided: 20
Macro Counts - Per Serving:
- Net Carbs: 0 g
- Calories: 575
- Protein: 24 g
- Fat Content: 51 g

Ingredients:
- 1 bone-in Standing rib roast (4 lb.) or (8 lb. - including bones)
- Sea salt (1.5 tbsp.)
- Black pepper (1 tsp.)
- Butter (.75 of 1 stick/6 tbsp. melted)
- Italian seasoning (2 tbsp.)
- Garlic (1 head/10-12 cloves/5-6 tsp. minced)

Preparation Technique:
1. Place the prime rib, fatty side up, onto a roasting pan fitted with a roasting rack. Sprinkle it using the sea salt and black pepper. Wait for one hour for the meat to acquire room temperature.
2. Set the oven at 450° Fahrenheit.
3. Stir the butter, Italian seasoning, and minced garlic. Pour the mixture over the prime rib and spread it evenly using a basting brush.
4. Roast the prime rib in the oven, uncovered, for 20-30 minutes, until the garlic on top is dark golden brown.
5. Tent the top of the prime rib with foil. Reduce the oven temperature to 350° Fahrenheit and continue roasting until the prime rib reaches your desired internal temperature

    For Rare: 110° Fahrenheit @ approximately 55 to 65 minutes

    For Med-Rare: 115° Fahrenheit @ approximately 60 to 70 minutes

    For Medium: 125 ° Fahrenheit @ approximately

65 to 80 minutes

Note: For medium-rare, it will take approximately an additional eight to nine minutes per pound of meat at 350° Fahrenheit after the first high-temp roast at 450° Fahrenheit. The above meat temperatures are not final temperatures, just the temperature to reach in the oven. The internal temperature will rise another 20 degrees in the next step.

6. Remove the prime rib from the oven. Wait for an additional 20 minutes before carving.

Ground Beef Cauliflower Lasagna

Servings Provided:6
Macro Counts - Per Serving - 1 cup each:
- Net Carbs: 10 g
- Calories: 386
- Protein: 28 g
- Fat Content: 24 g

Ingredients:
- Cauliflower (1 head - cut into florets)
- Olive oil (1 tbsp.)
- Ground beef (1 lb.)
- Onion (half of 1 large)
- Garlic cloves (2)
- Marinara sauce (1 cup)
- Diced tomatoes (14.5 oz. can)
- Fresh basil (.5 cup - chopped, divided)
- Mozzarella cheese (1 cup)
- Black pepper and sea salt (as desired)

Preparation Technique:
1. Chop or mince the onion and garlic. Shred the cheese.
2. Warm the oven at 400° Fahrenheit. Lightly grease a round 9-inch or square 9 by 9-inch casserole dish. Prepare the dish with a layer of aluminum foil.
3. Toss the cauliflower with the oil, sea salt, and black pepper. Roast it for 15 to 20 minutes, stirring halfway through, until crisp-tender.
4. Meanwhile, cook the onion in a skillet for 8 to10 minutes over medium-low heat, until it's slightly browned.
5. Add the ground beef and raise the temperature setting to medium-high. Cook for another eight to ten minutes until it's browned.
6. Stir in the garlic, marinara sauce, diced tomatoes, and half of the fresh basil, sea salt, and black pepper to taste. Cook it for two minutes, until heated thoroughly.

7. Pour the tomato meat sauce over the cauliflower. Sprinkle with shredded mozzarella cheese.
8. Bake it until the cheese bubbles (8 min.). Top with the remaining fresh basil ribbons.

Keto Burger Fat Bomb

Servings Provided: 20
Macro Counts - Per Serving:
- Net Carbs: 0 g
- Calories: 80
- Protein: 5 g
- Fat Content: 7 g

Ingredients:
- Ground beef (1 lb.)
- Garlic powder (.5 tsp.)
- Freshly ground black pepper & kosher salt (to your taste)
- Cold butter (2 tbsp./cut into 20 pieces)
- Cheddar (2 oz./cut into 20 pieces)
    For Serving:
- Lettuce leaves
- Thinly sliced tomatoes
- Mustard

Preparation Technique:
1. Warm the oven to 375° Fahrenheit. Lightly grease a mini muffin tin with a cooking oil spray. Mix the beef with salt, pepper, and garlic powder.
2. Press one teaspoon of the meat evenly into the bottom of each muffin tin cup. Add a tab of butter on top and press one teaspoon beef over the top.
3. Place a piece of cheddar on top of meat in each cup then press remaining beef over cheese to completely cover.
4. Bake it for about 15 minutes. Cool slightly.
5. Carefully release each burger from the tin. Serve with lettuce leaves, tomatoes, and mustard to your liking.

Skillet Steak - Nacho Style

Servings Provided:5
Macro Counts - Per Serving:
- Net Carbs: 6 g
- Calories: 385
- Protein: 19 g
- Fat Content: 31 g

Ingredients:

- Cauliflower (1.5 lb.)

- Turmeric (.5 tsp)

- Chili powder (1 tsp.)

- Butter (1 tbsp.)

- Beef round tip steak (8 oz.)

- Melted refined coconut oil (.33 cup)

- Shredded cheddar cheese (1 oz.)

- Shredded Monterey Jack cheese (1 oz.)
    Optional Garnishes:

- Sour cream (.33 cup)

- Canned - jalapeno slices (1 oz.)

- Avocado (approx. 5 oz.)

Preparation Technique:
1. Set the oven temperature at 400° Fahrenheit.
2. Prepare the cauliflower into chip-like shapes.
3. Combine the turmeric, chili powder, and coconut oil in a mixing dish.

4. Toss in the cauliflower and add it to a baking tin. Set the baking timer for 20 to 25 minutes.
5. Over med-high heat in a cast-iron skillet, add the butter. Cook until both sides of the meat is done, flipping just once. Let it rest for 5-10 minutes. Thinly slice and sprinkle with some pepper and salt.
6. When done, transfer the florets to the skillet and add the steak strips. Top it off with the cheese and bake for 5-10 more minutes.
7. Serve with your favorite garnish.
8. Count the carbs for the added garnishes.

Slow-Cooked Barbecue Meatloaf

Servings Provided:10
Macro Counts - Per Serving:
- Net Carbs: 3.49 g
- Calories: 369
- Protein: 26.95 g
- Fat Content: 22.49 g

Ingredients:
- Ground beef lean (2 lb.)
- Ground pork lean (1 lb.)
- Onion (.5 cup)
- Almond flour (.5 cup)
- Black pepper and salt (1 tsp.)
- Garlic powder (1 tsp.)
- Large eggs (2)
- Sugar-free BBQ sauce (1 cup)

Preparation Technique:
1. Finely chop the onion and combine it with the ground pork, ground beef, almond flour, salt, pepper, and garlic powder. Mix in the eggs until fully combined.
2. On a large sheet of tin foil, shape the mixture into a loaf (roughly 5 by 9 inches). Lift foil by edges and place in a six-quart slow cooker.
3. Set the slow cooker to low and cook for five to six hours.
4. In the last half hour of cooking, brush the top and sides with about ⅓ cup of barbecue sauce.
5. Use two serving forks to lift the meatloaf out of the cooker and onto a serving platter. Slice and serve with remaining barbecue sauce.

Chapter 8: Sauces - Gravy & Dressings

Keto Sauces

Avocado Mayonnaise

Servings Provided:4
Macro Counts - Per Serving:
- Net Carbs: 1 g
- Protein: 1 g
- Fat Content: 5 g

Ingredients:

- Ground cayenne pepper (.5 tsp.)

- Pinch of pink salt (1 pinch)

- Lime for juice (half of 1)

- Medium avocado (half of 1)

- Olive oil (.25 cup)

- Also Needed: Blender or food processor

Preparation Technique:
1. Dice the avocado. Combine the salt, cayenne, cilantro, avocado, and lime juice in the blender.
2. When smooth, stir in the oil - 1 tablespoon at a time - pulsing in between each addition.
3. It stores in the refrigerator for up to one week in a sealed glass bottle.

Easy Alfredo Sauce

Servings Provided:6
Macro Counts - Per Serving:
- Net Carbs: 3.8 g
- Calories: 531
- Protein: 10.3 g
- Fat Content: 53.8 g

Ingredients:
- Unsalted butter (.5 cup)
- Garlic (2 cloves)
- Heavy whipping cream (2 cups)
- Unchilled cream cheese (half of a 4 oz. pkg)
- Grated parmesan cheese (1.5 cups)
  Spices as Desired (1 pinch of each):
- Salt
- Ground nutmeg
- Ground white pepper

Preparation Technique:
1. Prepare a saucepan to melt the butter. Mince and add the garlic and sauté it for two minutes.
2. Pour in the cream and cream cheese.
3. Slowly add the parmesan until the sauce is thickened (5-7 min.)
4. Stir it thoroughly and serve with white pepper, nutmeg, and salt.

Enchilada Sauce

Servings Provided:
Macro Counts - Per Serving:
- Net Carbs: 5 g
- Calories: 198
- Protein: 2 g
- Fat Content: 18g

Ingredients:
- Butter (3 oz. - salted)
- Cayenne (.25 tsp.)
- Dried oregano (2 tsp.)
- Cumin, ground (3 tsp.)
- Coriander, ground (2 tsp.)
- Onion powder (2 tsp.)
- Erythritol (1.5 tbsp.)
- Tomato puree - only tomatoes and salt (12 oz.)
- Salt and pepper (.5 tsp.)

Preparation Technique:
1. Prepare a saucepan to melt the butter using the medium temperature setting.
2. Add each of the fixings - excluding the tomato puree- and sauté them for about three minutes.
3. Add in the puree and simmer the sauce for about five minutes. Thin with water as needed.
4. Use it immediately or store it in a heatproof jar. It remains delicious for about two weeks.

No-Cook Avocado Hollandaise

Servings Provided:4/1 cup each
Macro Counts - Per Serving:
- Net Carbs: 4 g
- Calories: 201
- Protein: 1 g
- Fat Content: 21 g

Ingredients:
- Ripe avocado (1 diced)
- Juice of 1 lemon
- Olive oil (.25 cup)
- Cayenne pepper (1 pinch)
- Kosher salt and freshly cracked black pepper

Preparation Technique:
1. In a blender or food processor, puree the avocado, lemon juice, and ⅓ cup water until combined.
2. With the motor running, add the olive oil in a slow stream and puree until the mixture has thickened with a creamy smooth texture.
3. Finish the hollandaise with cayenne, salt, and pepper. Serve it immediately.

Spicy Lemon Herb Sauce

Servings Provided:
Macro Counts - Per Serving:
- Net Carbs: 17 g
- Calories: 390
- Protein: 4 g
- Fat Content: 37 g

Ingredients:
- Shallot (1)
- Garlic (1 clove)
  Spices Needed (1 bunch of each):
- Parsley
- Mint
- Cilantro
- Lemons (2 zested & juiced)
- Olive oil (.33 cup)
- Salt (1 tsp.)
- Freshly cracked black pepper (2 tsp.)
- Red-pepper flakes (1 tsp.)

Preparation Technique:
1. Peel and roughly chop the shallot, parsley, mint, and cilantro. Juice the lemons and mince the garlic.
2. Pulse the garlic, herbs, shallot, and lemon zest in a food processor/blender.
3. Add the lemon juice, olive oil, pepper flakes, pepper, and salt to finish the sauce.
4. Transfer the sauce to an airtight container and refrigerate until ready to use. The sauce will keep for up to seven days.

Gravy Options

Brown Style Gravy

Servings Provided: 8
Macro Counts - Per Serving:
- Net Carbs: 0 g
- Calories: 56
- Protein: 1 g
- Fat Content: 6 g

Ingredients:
- Unsalted butter/butter substitute for dairy-free (.25 cup)
- Organic Vegetable Broth - ex. Pacific Foods (2 cups) or Turkey drippings (1 cup)
- Garlic powder (1 tsp.)
- Black pepper (.25 tsp.)
- Sea salt (1 tsp.)
- Xanthan gum (1 tsp.)
- Also Needed: 10-inch cast-iron skillet

Preparation Technique:
1. Warm the skillet to melt the butter using the medium temperature setting.
2. Whisk the xanthan gum, salt, and garlic pepper to add it into the skillet.
3. Pour in the vegetable broth and simmer.
4. Serve when it's thickened or save some for later.
5. Reheat it using the same process.

Creamy Mushroom Gravy Sauce

Servings Provided:
Macro Counts - Per Serving:
- Net Carbs: 4 g
- Calories: 165
- Protein: 3 g
- Fat Content: 14 g

Ingredients:
- Butter (1 tbsp.)
- Garlic (1 clove)
- Small onion (1)
- Salt (.5 tsp.)
- Pepper - ground (1 pinch)
- Mushrooms (7 oz.)
- Worcestershire Sauce (5 tsp.)
- Dijon mustard (1 tbsp.)
- Heavy cream (.5 cup)
- Fresh tarragon (2 tbsp.)

Preparation Technique:
1. Mince the garlic and thinly slice the onion and mushrooms. Chop the tarragon.
2. Prepare a saucepan using the high-temperature setting, add the butter, garlic, onion, salt, and pepper.
3. Sauté them until the onions are translucent.
4. Add the mushrooms and sauté them for three minutes before dropping the heat to the low setting.
5. Mix in the dijon mustard, Worcestershire sauce, and cream. Simmer it until the sauce thickens (10-15 min.).
6. Stir in the tarragon and serve.

Keto Onion Gravy For Meats

Servings Provided:8 @ 2 tbsp. each
Macro Counts - Per Serving:
- Net Carbs: 1 g
- Calories: 79
- Protein: 0 g
- Fat Content: 7 g

Ingredients:
- Water/pan drippings/meat stock (2 cups)
- Egg yolks (2 large)
- Onion (.5 cup)
- Butter or butter-flavored coconut oil (.25 cup)
- Pepper and salt (to your liking)
- Also Helpful: High-speed or stick blender

Preparation Technique:
1. Strain your pan drippings and add enough water or stock to make the two cups of liquid. Pour it into a saucepan and boil it to thicken (10 min.).
2. Add the onion and use the blender until it's pureed and continue cooking.
3. Take it from the burner. Pour and whisk about ¼ cup of the liquid into the yolks of the egg.
4. Whisk it all together until smooth and simmer until it's the way you like it.
5. Note: The gravy will thicken as it cools if you use the coconut oil, but the butter is better to thicken it. You can also add xanthan gum, coconut flour, or gelatin to thicken the gravy if you want it thicker (a great cheat technique).

Sausage Gravy

Servings Provided:4
Macro Counts - Per Serving:
- Net Carbs: 1.8 g
- Calories: 277
- Protein: 5.8 g
- Fat Content: 36 g

Ingredients:
- Breakfast sausage (4 oz.)
- Butter (2 tbsp.)
- Heavy cream (1 cup)
- Guar gum (.5 tsp.)
- Salt and pepper (as desired)

Preparation Technique:
1. Prepare the sausage in a skillet and set it aside.
2. Measure and add two tablespoons of butter to the grease. Once it's melted, add the cream and guar gum.
3. Stir and add the sausage to the mixture.
4. Continue stirring until it's thickened and serve it.

Tabasco Gravy

Servings Provided: 32
Macro Counts - Per Serving:
- Net Carbs: 1 g
- Calories: 90
- Protein: 3 g
- Fat Content: 8 g

Ingredients:
- Beef or bone broth (80 fl oz.)
- Bay leaves (2 fresh)
- Coconut cream - Rich & Extra-thick (0.5 cup/150 ml)
- Butter - unsalted (10 oz/284 g)
- Tabasco (about 2 dashes/2 tsp./9.4 g)
- Tamari (1 tbsp./16 g)
- Black pepper (2 tsp./2.8 g)
- Xanthan gum (1.66 tsp./2g)
- Kosher salt (as needed)

Preparation Technique:
1. Combine the heavy cream, broth, Tabasco, butter, bay leaves, and tamari in a saucepan. Gently simmer until the butter has melted, stirring often.
2. Cook for about 10-15 minutes until the sauce has reduced slightly.
3. Shake in the pepper and whisk in the xanthan gum to prevent lumps (1 tsp. at-a-time). Use a high-speed blender if desired.
4. Adjust the seasonings to our liking.

Chapter 9: Desserts

Keto Pie Crust

Servings Provided: 10
Macro Counts - Per Serving:
- Net Carbs: 1.8 g
- Calories: 187
- Protein: 3.7 g
- Fat Content: 12.7 g

Ingredients:
- Salt (.25 tsp.)
- Butter - melted (.25 cup)

Preparation Method:
1. Whisk the salt, sweetener, and flour in a mixing container. Fold in the melted butter to form coarse crumbs.
2. Dump it into a pie plate and press it firmly to the sides and bottom. Prick it using a toothpick or fork.
3. For unfilled Crust: Bake 325° Fahrenheit for about 20 minutes.
4. For filled Crust: Pre-bake it for 10-12 minutes before adding the fixings. Cover the edges to avoid over-browning.

Brownie in a Mug

Servings Provided: 1
Macro Counts - Per Serving:
- Net Carbs: 5 g
- Calories: 310
- Protein: 35 g
- Fat Content: 15 g

Ingredients:

- Granulated sweetener (1 tbsp.)

- Eggs (2)

- Heavy cream (1 tbsp.)

- Protein powder (1 scoop)

Preparation Technique:
1. You will love this one.
2. Add the eggs, cream sweetener, and protein powder into the chosen mug. Thoroughly stir the mixture.
3. Place the cup in the microwave for one minute. Remove with caution and devour it.

Cheesecake Mocha Bars

Servings Provided: 16
Macro Counts - Per Serving:
- Net Carbs: 3.24 g
- Calories: 232
- Protein: 6.1 g
- Fat Content: 21.2 g

Ingredients:
   Brownie Layer:

- Vanilla extract (2 tsp.)

- Unsalted butter (6 tbsp.)

- Large eggs (3)

- Almond flour (1.5 cups)

- Hershey's Baking Cocoa or your preference (.5 cup)

- Erythritol (1 cup)

- Salt (.5 tsp.)

- Instant coffee (.5 tbsp.)

- Baking powder (1 tsp.)
   Cream Cheese Layer:

- Erythritol (.5 cup)

- Large egg (1)

- Softened cream cheese (1 lb.)

- Vanilla extract (1 tsp.)

- Also Needed: 8x8-inch baking pan

Preparation Technique:
1. Set the oven temperature to 350° Fahrenheit. Lightly grease or spray the pan.
2. Combine the wet fixings starting with the vanilla and butter. Next, mix in the eggs.
3. In another container, combine the dry ingredients and whisk with the wet fixings. Set aside ¼ cup of the batter for later. Pour the mixture into the pan.
4. Mix the cream cheese (room temperature) with the remainder of the fixings for the second layer. Spread it on the sheet of brownies.
5. Use the reserved batter as the last layer (will be thin). Bake for 30 to 35 minutes. When cooled, slice the cheesecake bars, and enjoy.

Chia Bars

Servings Provided:14
Macro Counts - Per Serving:
- Net Carbs: 1.5 g
- Calories: 121
- Protein: 2.5 g
- Fat Content: 11 g

Ingredients:

- Toasted almonds (.5 cup)

- Coconut oil (divided - 1 tbsp. (+) 1 tsp.)

- Erythritol (4 tbsp. - divided)

- Butter (2 tbsp.)

- Heavy cream (.25 tsp.)

- Liquid stevia (.25 tsp.)

- Vanilla extract (1.5 tsp.)

- Unsweetened & shredded coconut flakes (.5 cup)

- Chia seeds (.25 cup)

- Coconut cream (.5 cup)

- Coconut flour (2 tbsp.)

- Also Needed: Food Processor

Preparation Technique:

1. Add the toasted almonds into the food processor and pulse until crumbly.
2. Toss in one tablespoon of the coconut oil and two tablespoons of the erythritol. Continue processing

until you have almond butter. (Now you have another new usable product.)

3. Warm a pan and add the butter, heavy cream, erythritol, stevia, and vanilla. Stir until they're bubbly and fold in the almond butter. Stir to blend.

4. In a blender, grind the chia seeds to make a powdery mix. In another pan, toast the coconut flakes and mix with the chia seeds. Melt the coconut cream in a separate skillet.

5. Now, combine all of the fixings and add the melted coconut cream, flour, and coconut oil. Store in the fridge for one hour.

6. When it's ready, slice into squares and store in the refrigerator.

Chocolate Lava Cake

Servings Provided: 4
Macro Counts - Per Serving:
- Net Carbs: 3 g
- Calories: 189
- Protein: 8 g
- Fat Content: 17 g

Ingredients:

- Unsweetened cocoa powder (.5 cup)

- Melted butter (.25 cup)

- Eggs (4)

- Sugar-free chocolate sauce (.25 cup)

- Sea salt (.5 tsp.)

- Ground cinnamon (.5 tsp.)

- Pure vanilla extract (1 tsp.)

- Stevia (.25 cup)

- Also Needed: Ice cube tray & 4 ramekins

Preparation Technique:
1. Pour one tablespoon of the chocolate sauce into four of the tray slots and freeze.
2. Warm up the oven to 350⁰ Fahrenheit. Lightly grease the ramekins with butter or a spritz of oil.
3. Mix the salt, cinnamon, cocoa powder, and stevia until combined. Whisk in the eggs – one at a time. Stir in the melted vanilla extract and butter.

4. Fill each of the ramekins halfway and add one of the frozen chocolates. Cover the rest of the container with the cake batter.
5. Bake for 13-14 minutes. When they're set, place on a wire rack to cool for about five minutes. Remove and put on a serving dish.
6. Enjoy by slicing its molten center.

Cinnamon Twists

Servings Provided:10 twists
Macro Counts - Per Serving:
- Net Carbs: 3.6 g
- Calories: 174
- Protein: 5.7 g
- Fat Content: 14.7 g

Ingredients:
The Dough:
- Coconut flour (.25 cup)
- Almond flour (.5 cup)
- Baking powder (1 tsp.)
- Swerve sweetener - powdered (.25 cup)
- Shredded mozzarella cheese - part-skim(1.5 cups)
- Butter (5 tbsp.) + melted (2 tbsp.)
- Egg (1 large)
- Vanilla extract (.5 tsp.)
- Swerve sweetener - granulated (2 tsp.)
- Cinnamon (1 tsp.)
   The Glaze:
- Swerve sweetener - powdered (2 tbsp.)
- Vanilla extract (.25 tsp.)
- Water

Preparation Technique:

1. Warm the oven to 350° Fahrenheit.
2. Cover a large baking mat with parchment paper.
3. Combine the sweetener, baking powder, almond flour, and coconut flour.
4. Melt the cheese and butter over low heat in a large saucepan until it can be stirred together. Whisk and add the vanilla and egg. Stir in the almond flour mixture to form the dough (low-temperature setting). Dump it onto the countertop and knead it together.
5. Cover the dough using a layer of parchment baking paper. Roll out to a 10 by 10-inch square. Brush the dough using about half of the melted butter.
6. Whisk the swerve and cinnamon, dusting about ⅔ of it over the dough.
7. Fold the dough in half and cut into ten strips with a sharp knife.
8. Hold both ends of one strip and twist gently in opposite directions two or three times. Lay twists on the prepared baking sheet and brush with the rest of the melted butter and cinnamon sugar.
9. Set the timer to bake for 15 minutes.
10. Prep the Glaze: Mix the vanilla extract, powdered sweetener, and enough water to achieve a drizzling consistency.
11. Add the glaze over the cooled cinnamon twists and serve as desired.

Coconut Chia Bars

Servings Provided: 6 bars
Macro Counts - Per Serving:
- Net Carbs: 3.5 g
- Calories: 164
- Protein: 4 g
- Fat Content: 14 g

Ingredients

- Chia seeds (4 tbsp.)

- Water (.5 cup)

- Coconut oil (1 tbsp.

- Confectioners Swerve (1 tbsp.)

- Vanilla extract (.25 tsp.)

- Shredded dried coconut meat – unsweetened (1 cup)

- Cashews (.5 cup)

- Also Needed: 9 x 9 cookie sheet

Preparation Technique:
1. Set the oven temperature to 350⁰ Fahrenheit.
2. Soak the seeds 15 minutes until gel-like, and mix with the coconut, oil, swerve, and vanilla extract. Lastly, add in the cashews.
3. Line the mixture, using parchment paper, onto the baking tin. Press until it is about a 3/4-inch thickness, and bake for 45 minutes.
4. Slice into six bars and enjoy!

Dark Chocolate Brownies

Servings Provided: 16
Macro Counts - Per Serving:
- Net Carbs: 4 g
- Calories: 76
- Protein: 3 g
- Fat Content: 8 g

Ingredients:

- Cream cheese (6 tbsp.)

- Eggs (3)

- Coconut oil (3 tbsp.)

- Cocoa powder (heaping 2 tbsp.)

- Almond flour (.25 cup)

- Coconut flour (.25 cup)

- Baking soda (.25 tbsp.)

- Truvia (9 packets)

- Almond milk (.5 cup)

- Vanilla extract (1 tsp.)

- Salt (1 pinch)

Preparation Technique:
1. Heat the oven to reach 375º Fahrenheit.
2. Lightly spritz the baking tin with cooking oil spray.
3. Whisk the eggs, cream cheese, milk, coconut oil, and vanilla extract.

4. In another container, mix the dry fixings (almond flour, cocoa powder, coconut flour, Truvia, baking soda, and a pinch of salt).
5. Combine everything and scoop into the cake pan. Bake for about half an hour and chill before serving.

Gingerbread – Slow Cooked

Servings Provided: 10
Macro Counts - Per Serving:
- Net Carbs: 8.6 g
- Calories: 223
- Protein: 9.1 g
- Fat Content: 24.8 g

Ingredients:

- Almond/sunflower seed flour (2.25 cups)

- Coconut flour (2 tbsp.)

- Salt (.25 tsp.)

- Ground cloves (.5 tsp.)

- Swerve sweetener (.75 cup)

- Ground ginger (1.5 tbsp.)

- Dark cocoa powder (1 tbsp.)

- Ground cinnamon (.5 tsp.)

- Baking powder (2 tsp.)

- Large eggs (4)

- Melted butter (.5 cup)

- Fresh lemon juice (1 tbsp.)

- Water or almond milk (.66 cup)

- Vanilla extract (1 tsp.)

- Recommended Size: Six quarts

Preparation Technique:

1. Spritz the cooker with some cooking oil spray.
2. Whisk salt, all of the flour, cloves, baking powder, ginger, cinnamon, sweetener, and cocoa powder in a large mixing container.
3. Blend in the eggs, melted butter, almond milk or water, vanilla extract, and lemon juice.
4. Empty the batter into the slow cooker and cook until set - approximately 2.5 to 3 hours.
5. Garnish as desired and enjoy, but count those carbs.

Individual Strawberry Cheesecakes

Servings Provided: 4
Macro Counts - Per Serving:
- Net Carbs: 9 g
- Calories: 489
- Protein: 8 g
- Fat Content: 47 g

Ingredients:
   The Crust:
- Almond flour (.5 cup)
- Melted butter/coconut oil (3 tbsp.)
- Sugar substitute – your preference (.25 cup) or Maple syrup
   The Filling:

- Sugar substitute (3 tbsp.) or use Grade B maple syrup

- Strawberries (6)

- Cream cheese (8 oz.)

- Sour cream (.33 cup)

- Pure vanilla extract (.5 tsp.)
   The Garnish:

- Strawberries (4)

- Fresh mint leaves

Preparation Technique:
1. Combine the crust fixings in a mixing bowl. Blend well and divide it into four small ramekins. Gently press with your fingers.
2. Prepare the filling in a food processor. Pulse until creamy smooth.

3. Divide it over the crust of each one and chill for an hour or until it's set.
4. Garnish with another berry if desired and serve. (Add the carbs for any added garnishes.)

Lemon Cake

Servings Provided:8
Macro Counts - Per Serving:
- Net Carbs: 5.2 g
- Calories: 350
- Protein: 7.6 g
- Fat Content: 33 g

Ingredients:

- Coconut flour (.5 cup)

- Baking powder (2 tsp.)

- Almond flour (1.5 cups)

- Swerve (or) Pyure A-P (3 tbsp.)

- Optional: Xanthan gum (.5 tsp.)

- Whipping cream (.5 cup)

- Melted butter (.5 cup)

- Zest & juice (2 lemons)

- Eggs (2)
    Ingredients for the Topping:
- Pyure all-purpose/Swerve (3 tbsp.)

- Lemon juice (2 tbsp.)

- Boiling water (.5 cup)

- Melted butter (2 tbsp.)

- Suggested: 2-4-quart slow cooker

Preparation Technique:

1. For the Cake: Mix the dry ingredients in a container. Whisk the egg, lemon juice and zest, butter, and whipping cream. Combine all of the fixings and mix well. Scoop out the dough into the prepared slow cooker.
2. For the Topping: Mix all of the topping ingredients in a container and empty over the batter in the cooker.
3. Place the lid on the cooker for two to three hours on the high setting.
4. Serve warm with some fresh fruit or whipped cream.

Lemon Custard Tarts

Yields Provided: 2 servings
Macro Counts For Each Serving:

- Net Carbs: 2 g
- Calories: 954
- Protein: 17 g
- Fat Content: 95 g

Ingredients - The Crust:

- Unsalted melted butter (3 tbsp.)

- Almond meal (.75 cup)

- *Optional*: Dried lavender flowers (.5 tsp.)

- Sugar-free Vanilla bean sweetener syrup – ex. Torani (1 tbsp.)
  The Filling:

- Freshly squeezed lemon juice (.5 cup)

- Large egg yolks (4)

- Grated zest of a lemon (3)

- Melted unsalted butter (.5 cup)

- Sugar-free vanilla syrup/your choice (.25 to .5 cup)

- *Also Needed:* 2 crème Brule dishes – 4.5-inch x 1.25 thick

Preparation Technique:
1. Warm the oven to reach 375° Fahrenheit.
2. Lightly spritz the dishes using ghee or butter.
3. *Prepare the Crust*: If you're using the flowers, grind them into fine dust with a mortar and pestle. Mix it with three tablespoons of melted butter and almond flour. Press into the bottom of the two dishes.
4. Bake until the tops start browning (10 min.). Transfer to the counter to cool.
5. *Prepare the Filling*: Use a food processor or blender to mix the sweetener, lemon juice, egg yolks, lemon zest, and rest of the butter. Scoop into a saucepan (med-low) and simmer about 15 minutes or until it's pudding-like.
6. When ready, pour the filling over the two crusts.
7. Secure a layer of plastic wrap over each one and refrigerate overnight.

Mocha Pudding Cake – Slow Cooked

Servings Provided: 6
Macro Counts - Per Serving:
- Net Carbs: 3.8 g
- Calories: 414
- Protein: 9.3 g
- Fat Content: 30 g

Ingredients:

- Coconut oil spray or butter – for the cooker

- Finely chopped unsweetened chocolate (2 oz.)

- Butter – large chunks (.75 cup)

- Heavy cream (.5 cup)

- Vanilla extract (1 tsp.)

- Instant coffee crystals (2 tbsp.)

- Almond flour (1.33 cup)

- Unsweetened cocoa powder (4 tbsp.)

- Salt (.125 tsp.)

- Large eggs (5)

- Stevia erythritol granulated sweetener (.66 cup)

- Optional: Low-carb whipped cream/ice cream

- Recommended: 4-6-quart slow cooker

Preparation Technique:
1. Grease the cooker with butter/spray.
2. Using the medium heat setting on the stovetop, melt

the unsweetened chocolate and butter in a small pan.
Whisk occasionally. Take it off of the burner and cool.
3. Whisk the heavy cream, vanilla extract, and coffee crystals in a small container.
4. Mix the cocoa, flour, and salt in another dish.
5. Whip the eggs using a mixer (high-speed). Slowly add the sweetener when thickened. Beat on the high setting for about five minutes.
6. Slowly, on the low setting, use the mixer to combine the unsweetened chocolate mixture and butter – adding it to the cake mixture.
7. Fold in the flour, salt, and cocoa mixture. Blend (medium speed), and add the coffee, cream, and vanilla ingredients.
8. Add the batter to the prepared slow cooker, and place a paper towel over the slow cooker top to absorb the moisture.
9. Secure the lid and cook using the low setting for 2.5 to 3.5 hours (4-quart cooker) or 2-3 hours (6-quart cooker).
10. Test for doneness in the center at 160° Fahrenheit. The center will be a soft soufflé consistency with an outer cake-like appearance.
11. Enjoy, but remember to count the extra carbs.

Pistachio Dark Chocolate Tart

Servings Provided: 4
Macro Counts - Per Serving:
- Net Carbs: 6 g
- Calories: 490
- Protein: 13 g
- Fat Content: 46 g

Ingredients:
   The Crust:

- Coconut flour (1 cup)

- Flaxseed meal (.25 cup)

- Sugar substitute – your preference (3 tbsp. or to taste)

- Butter (.5 cup)

- Egg whites (4)
   The Filling:

- Raw unsweetened cocoa powder (.5 cup)

- Heavy cream (1 cup)

- Gelatin powder (2.5 tsp.

- Sugar substitute (.25 cup or to taste)

- Pure vanilla extract (1 tsp.)

- Sliced pistachios (.25 cup)

Preparation Technique::
1. Heat the oven at 375° Fahrenheit. Prepare a pie pan or small tart pan with a spritz of cooking oil spray.

2. Combine the crust fixings in a food processor. Pulse
   until well mixed. Press into the prepared pan/pans.
   Bake for 15 minutes.
3. When it is ready, put the pan on a rack to cool.
4. Prepare the filling by combining all of the components
   except for the pistachios into a blender. Mix well until
   it's creamy.
5. Dump the mixture to the prepared crust/crusts. Cover
   the pie with a sheet of plastic wrap. Place it in the
   fridge for about 2 hours. It should be firm.
6. When ready to serve, add the sliced pistachios.

Pumpkin Bars with Cream Cheese Frosting

Servings Provided: 16
Macro Counts - Per Serving:
- Net Carbs: 2 g
- Calories: 139
- Protein: 3 g
- Fat Content: 13 g

Ingredients:

- Large eggs (2)

- Coconut oil (.25 cup)

- Pumpkin puree (1 cup)

- Cream cheese (2 oz.)

- Almond flour (1 cup)

- Gluten-free baking powder (2 tsp.)

- Erythritol sweetener blend (.66 cups)

- Pumpkin pie spice (1 tsp.)

- Sea salt (.5 tsp.)

- Vanilla extract (1 tsp.)

  The Frosting:

- Powdered erythritol (.5 cup)

- Optional: Heavy cream (1 tbsp.)

- Softened cream cheese (6 oz.)

- Vanilla extract (1 tsp.)

- Also Needed: 9 x 9 baking pan

Preparation Method:
1. Warm the oven until it reaches 350° Fahrenheit. Cover the baking pan with parchment paper.
2. In a double boiler or microwave, melt the coconut oil and cream cheese.
3. Combine the vanilla, eggs, cream cheese, and puree using a hand mixer until smooth (medium-speed).
4. Whisk the dry fixings (salt, pie spice, baking powder, sweetener, and flour).
5. Mix all the ingredients with the mixer until just combined and pour into the pan.
6. Bake for 20 to 30 minutes. Cool completely.
7. Prepare the frosting with each of the ingredients when the bars are cooled. If it's too thick, just add a little cream or milk.
8. Slice into 16 equal portions.

Spice Cakes

Servings Provided: 12
Macro Counts - Per Serving:
- Net Carbs: 3 g
- Calories: 277
- Protein: 6 g
- Fat Content: 27 g

Ingredients:

- Salted butter (.5 cup)

- Erythritol (.75 cup)

- Eggs (4 - divided)

- Vanilla extract (1 tsp.)

- Ground cloves (.25 tsp.)

- Baking powder (2 tsp.)

- Allspice (.5 tsp.)

- Nutmeg (.5 tsp.

- Almond flour (2 cups)

- Cinnamon (.5 tsp.)

- Ginger (.5 tsp.)

- Water (5 tbsp.)

- Also Needed: Cupcake tray

Preparation Technique:
1. Warm the oven temperature to 350° Fahrenheit. Prepare the baking tray with liners (12).

2. Mix the butter and erythritol with a hand mixer. Once it's smooth, combine with two eggs and the vanilla. Add the rest of the eggs and mix well.
3. Grind the clove to a fine powder and add with the rest of the spices. Whisk into the mixture. Stir in the baking powder and almond flour. Blend in the water. When the batter is smooth, add to the prepared tin.
4. Bake for 15 minutes. Enjoy any time.

Zucchini Bread

Servings Provided:12
Macro Counts - Per Serving:
- Net Carbs: 13.8 g
- Calories: 174
- Protein: 5 g
- Fat Content: 15.7 g

Ingredients:

- Almond flour (1 cup)

- Cinnamon (2 tsp.)

- Coconut flour (.33 cup)

- Baking powder (1.5 tsp.)

- Optional: xanthan gum (.5 tsp.)

- Salt (.5 tsp.)

- Baking soda (.5 tsp.)

- Softened coconut oil or butter (.33 cup)

- Eggs (3)

- Vanilla (2 tsp.)

- Pyure all-purpose (.5 cup)

- Shredded zucchini as desired

- Chopped pecans or walnuts (.5 cup)

- Also Needed: 4 by 8 silicone bread pan

Preparation Technique:

1. Combine the coconut and almond flour, salt, baking soda, and powder, cinnamon, and xanthan gum. Set aside for now.
2. Mix the oil, eggs, vanilla, and sugar in another dish. Combine the fixings.
3. Blend in the nuts and shredded zucchini. Scoop the batter into the prepared bread pan.
4. Arrange the cooker on the top rack (or on crunched up aluminum foil balls). You want it at least ½-inch from the bottom of the slow cooker.
5. Put the top on the cooker and prepare for three hours using the high-temperature setting.
6. Cool, wrap in foil, and place in the fridge. It is best when refrigerated.

Chapter 10: 16-Day Meal Plan

Each of these recipes has the net carbs per serving posted. You will see how flexible the plan is when you look at how easy it is to use just the recipes in this cookbook with the following two weeks and two days as a bonus into the third week. The plan includes three meals, snacks, or desserts.

The meals are planned, so you still have flexibility in your eating patterns with extra carbs to use as desired. Even on the strictest diet plan, most of these recipes should be just what the doctor ordered. Calculate how many carbs you are allowed each day and add some healthy snacks or sides to these totals. It's all up to you; just track everything.

Day 1:

Breakfast: Breakfast Skillet: 7.1 g

Lunch: Egg Drop Soup: 3 g

Dinner: Pan-Fried Fried Cod: 1 g

Dessert or Snack: Lemon Cake: 5.2 g

Day 2:

Breakfast: Eggs Benedict Quiche: 3.8 g

Lunch: Greek Meatball Salad: 2 g

Dinner: Creamy Onion Chicken: 3 g

Dessert or Snack: Pistachio Dark Chocolate Tart: 6 g

Day 3:

Breakfast: Sausage & Cheese Omelet Roll: 3.45 g

Lunch: Zoodles & White Clam Sauce: 7 g

Dinner: Kalua Pork & Cabbage: 4 g

Dessert or Snack: Spice Cakes: 3 g

Day 4:

Breakfast: Sugar-Free Krispy Kreme™ Doughnuts: 1.3 g

Lunch: 2 Ingredient Keto Pasta: 3 g &Greek Chopped Salad: 2 g

Dinner: Cheeseburger Calzone: 3 g

Dessert or Snack: Mocha Pudding Cake – Slow Cooked: 3.8 g

Day 5:

Breakfast: Mini Bacon & Kale Frittatas: 4.07 g

Lunch: Cabbage Roll 'Unstuffed' Soup: 3 g

Dinner: Chicken Mozzarella & Pesto Casserole: 3 g

Dessert or Snack: Lemon Custard Tarts: 2 g

Day 6:

Breakfast: Pumpkin Spice Egg Loaf: 2.6 g

Lunch: Kiwi & Feta Chicken Salad: 13 g

Dinner: Mahi-Mahi Fillets: 0 g

Dessert or Snack: Cinnamon Twists: 3.6 g

Day 7:

Breakfast: Southwestern Cauliflower Breakfast Pizza: 2.6 g

Lunch: Creamy Salmon Pasta: 3 g

Dinner: Pork Kebabs: 3.3 g

Dessert or Snack: Gingerbread – Slow Cooked: 8.6 g

Day 8:

Breakfast: Cocoa Waffles: 3.4 g

Lunch: Philly Cheesesteak: 6 g

Dinner: Kung Pao Chicken: 4 g

Dessert or Snack: Chocolate Lava Cake: 3

Day 9:

Breakfast: Bacon & Egg Breakfast Muffins: 0.4 g

Lunch: Chili Delight - No-Beans: 5 g

Dinner: Shrimp Alfredo: 6.5 g

Dessert or Snack: Pumpkin Bars With Cream Cheese Frosting: 2 g

Day 10:

Breakfast: Chocolate Loaf: 2.32 g

Lunch: Shrimp & Fish Roe Salad Sandwiches: 2 g

Dinner: Kung Pao Chicken: 4 g

Dessert or Snack: Individual Strawberry Cheesecakes: 9 g

Day 11:

Breakfast: BLT Wrap For Brunch: 2 g

Lunch: Steak Salad: 1.5 g

Dinner: Chicken Enchilada Bowl: 6 g

Dessert or Snack: Brownie in a Mug: 5 g

Day 12:

Breakfast: Pigs In Pancakes: 3.04 g

Lunch: Curried-Style Fish Stew: 8 g

Dinner: Crunchy Fish and Chaffle Bites: 1.3 g

Dessert or Snack: Cheesecake Mocha Bars: 3.24 g

Day 13:

Breakfast: Green Buttered Eggs: 2.5 g

Lunch: Tuna Salad & Chives: 1 g

Dinner: Lemon Parsley Buttered Chicken - Slow Cooked: 1 g

Dessert or Snack: Zucchini Bread: 13.8 g

Day 14:

Breakfast: Sausage Gravy & Biscuits: 2 g

Lunch: Asiago Tomato Soup: 8.75 g

Dinner: Skillet Steak - Nacho Style: 6 g

Dessert or Snack: Dark Chocolate Brownies: 4 g

Day 15:

Breakfast: Bacon & Brie Frittata: 1.7 g

Lunch: Jar Salad: 4 g

Dinner: Lemon Butter Scallops: 5 g

Dessert or Snack: Coconut Chia Bars: 3.5 g

Day 16:

Breakfast: Peanut Butter Protein Bars: 3 g

Lunch: Gluten-Free - Vegan Zucchini 'Meatballs': 1.1 g

Dinner: Italian Parmesan Chicken Meatballs: 3 g &

Keto Spaghetti Sauce: 2 g

Dessert or Snack: Brownie in a Mug: 5 g

Now, you see how easy it is to go Keto; make these your new favorite recipes!

Of course, there are plenty more recipes, just like these!

Conclusion

I hope you have thoroughly enjoyed each segment of your personal copy of *Easy Everyday Keto*. I hope it was informative and provided you with all of the tools you need to achieve your goals, whatever they may be.

Remember to skip the highest ranks of GPS – grains, potatoes, and sugar.
Focus on veggies, fats, and proteins. Visit a restaurant that offers a healthy salad bar, seafood spreads, carving stations, and vegetable platters. You can usually find butter, olive oil, sour cream, and cheese in plentiful supply.

Use a smaller plate. Play a mind game and fill a small plate instead of a larger one. Try it, this really works.

Make Wise Drink Decisions: The best choice is water, tea, coffee, or sparkling water. Decaf coffee or herbal tea is another excellent option. If alcohol is your craving, choose dry wine, champagne, or light beer. Also, consider spirits – straight or with a bit of club soda.

Choose Dessert Wisely: If you are still hungry, try to have another cup of tea or a cheese platter. Have a portion of berries with heavy cream. What about some cream in your coffee?

Take your time. Enjoy your time spent with the conversation of a friend or family member. Drink your water and sip your tea or coffee. Enjoy and feel satisfied!

You may experience some headaches, fatigue, or nausea, which is sometimes called 'induction flu.' As you remove the carbs, your potassium and sodium (vital electrolytes) are also removed. Taking a supplement will help with these issues.

Sodium Supplements: You should receive at least one to two grams of extra sodium daily. Some of the pros accomplish this with bouillon cubes. Sea Salt is a great option used in your diet plan. You should receive 3000 to 5000 mg of sodium daily.

Potassium Supplement: You can become low in potassium in the short-term because of the vomiting and diarrhea that could go along with your early stages to the keto plan. Natural potassium can also be received through milk, whole grains, bananas, veggies, peas, and beans. It is recommended to take supplements because potassium also leaves your body with salt. As part of your well-prepared meal plan, you should receive 3000 to 4000 mg of potassium daily.

Magnesium Supplement: For magnesium, 300-500 mg is an initial recommendation. Muscle cramps are your best indicator of depletion.

You may not need these supplements, but it's always a good idea to know which ones would help should you experience any discomfort during the progression of the ketogenic diet and its restrictions.

Finally, if you found this book useful in any way, a review on Amazon is always appreciated!

Find us on Instagram, where we share contents and photos about the book and the Ketogenic world:

easy.everydayketo
Andrew Shelby
https://www.instagram.com/easy.everydayketo

Index For The Recipes:

10. Roasted Cauliflower With Blue Cheese Sauce & Bacon
11. Spinach Salmon Roulade
12. Sushi

Smoothies For A Quick Refreshing Snack - Meal Or Appetizer:
13. Almond Lover Smoothie
14. Banana Bread & Blueberry Smoothie
15. Keto Avocado-Raspberry Smoothie
16. Strawberry Almond Smoothies

Chapter 6: Seafood & Poultry Specialties

Seafood Favorites

1. Blue Crabs With Lime - Chipotle & Brown Butter Sauce
2. Broiled Oyster With Spicy Sauce
3. Cajun Trinity Keto Crab Cakes
4. Chaffles & Prawns With Toppings
5. Cioppino Italian Seafood Stew - Gluten-Free
6. Crunchy Fish and Chaffle Bites
7. Lemon Butter Scallops
8. Mahi-Mahi Fillets
9. Pan-Fried Fried Cod
10. Shrimp Alfredo
11. Shrimp & Bacon Risotto
12. Tuna Fritter

Poultry Options
1. Asparagus-Stuffed Chicken
2. Bacon-Wrapped Chicken - Air Fryer
3. Chicken Enchilada Bowl
4. Chicken Mozzarella & Pesto Casserole
5. Chicken Parmesan Meatballs
6. Chicken Tenders - Chick-fil-A Copycat
7. Creamy Onion Chicken
8. *Kung Pao Chicken*

Chapter 9: Desserts
1. Keto Pie Crust
2. Brownie in a Mug
3. Cheesecake Mocha Bars
4. Chia Bars
5. Chocolate Lava Cake
6. Cinnamon Twists
7. Coconut Chia Bars
8. Dark Chocolate Brownies
9. Gingerbread – Slow Cooked
10. Individual Strawberry Cheesecakes
11. Lemon Cake
12. Lemon Custard Tarts
13. Mocha Pudding Cake – Slow Cooked
14. Pistachio Dark Chocolate Tart
15. Pumpkin Bars With Cream Cheese Frosting
16. Spice Cakes
17. Zucchini Bread